To Chuck

...the body's pain and the pain on the streets
are not the same   but you can learn
from the edges that blur   O you who love clear edges
more than anything   watch the edges that blur

                    -- Adrienne Rich
                     "Contradictions: Tracking
                    Poems"

If one is sick of sickness
then one is not sick.

                    -- Lao Tsu
                    Tao Te Ching LXXI

Current Clinical Strategies

Manual of HIV/AIDS Therapy

Laurence Peiperl, MD

Program in Primary Care Internal Medicine
University of California, San Francisco
San Francisco General Hospital

Paul D. Chan, MD
Associate Editor

Acknowledgements
The author is grateful to the following physicians for editorial guidance:

Michael Clement, MD

Assistant Professor of Medicine, University of California, San Francisco
Medical Director, AIDS Outpatient Clinic, San Francisco General Hospital

Mark A. Jacobson, MD

Assistant Professor of Medicine, University of California, San Francisco
Director of Clinical Research, AIDS Div., San Francisco General Hospital

John D. Stansell, MD

Assistant Professor of Medicine, University of California, San Francisco
Director, Inpatient AIDS Service, San Francisco General Hospital

Molly Cooke, MD

Associate Professor of Medicine, University of California, San Francisco

Allen L. Gifford, MD

Department of Medicine, University of California, San Francisco

Cynthia Fenton, MD

Chief Medical Resident, San Francisco General Hospital

Paul A. Volberding, MD

Professor of Medicine, University of California, San Francisco
Director, AIDS Division, San Francisco General Hospital

Thanks also to **Dan Kilpatrick**
University of California, San Francisco, Department of Medicine

Preface

This book was written to educate and assist the many attending physicians, house officers and medical students who are involved in the day-to-day care of adult patients with HIV disease. Epidemiology, natural history, and clinical management of HIV infection are discussed in the first section. Infectious diseases that occur commonly in patients with AIDS are covered in detail in subsequent chapters. Additionally, diseases that are not unique to AIDS, but that differ in the setting of HIV infection from their usual presentation, are included in the last section. Neoplastic disorders such as Kaposi's sarcoma and lymphoma are covered as they occur in the differential diagnosis of various AIDS related disorders.

Current Clinical Strategies Publishing International
9550 Warner Ave., Suite 350
Fountain Valley, California, USA 92708-2822
Phone: 714-965-9400
FAX of Voice mail: 714-965-9401

Printed in USA

ISBN 1-881528-01-4

Transmission, Prevention, and Primary Care of HIV Infection

I. Introduction (1,2)

Acquired immunodeficiency syndrome (AIDS) is a viral disease caused by the human immunodeficiency virus (HIV). The virus is spread though sexual contact; through contact with blood, blood products, or other bodily fluids (including intravenous drug use); or perinatally from mother to infant. The primary feature of the disease AIDS is a defect in cell-mediated immunity, leading to multiple opportunistic infections and neoplasms.

By the beginning of 1992, over 200,000 cases of AIDS and 130,000 deaths from AIDS have been reported in the United States. The World Health Organization estimates that the number of persons infected with HIV is 10 million, and this number is likely to double by the year 2000.

Of the estimated one million persons infected with HIV in the United States, approximately 20% have AIDS by the current Centers for Disease Control (CDC) definition. The CDC defines AIDS as a condition in which an HIV infected individual contracts any of a list of opportunistic infections, neoplasms, or severe symptoms indicative of severe immunodeficiency (2). It is estimated that an additional 12% would qualify for a diagnosis of AIDS under a revised (but un-adopted) policy that would extend the definition of AIDS to any individual with HIV infection and a T-helper cell count (T4 count, CD4 count) of less than 200 CD4-positive cells per microliter.

Approximately 2% of the total number of AIDS cases in the U.S. have occurred in children. Of the adult cases, 55% have occurred in homosexual or bisexual men, 23% in intravenous drug users (IVDU's), and 6% in men with a history of both homosexual sex and intravenous drug use. Heterosexual contact with a person at high risk of HIV infection was the only risk factor in 6% of cases, blood transfusion in 2%, and clotting factor use (hemophilia or other coagulation disorder) in 1%. No risk factor was determined in 4%.

The proportion of cases among women and minorities is increasing. Over the past two years, 12% of U.S. AIDS diagnoses occurred in women, 31% in Blacks, and 17% in Hispanics. The proportion of cases attributed to heterosexual transmission is also increasing steadily.

II. Transmission of HIV infection

Routes of Transmission of HIV:

Sexual transmission: Receptive anal intercourse (homosexual or heterosexual) with an infected partner carries a high risk of transmitting the virus. Male-to-female and female-to-male transmission can occur during vaginal intercourse. However, the correct use of condoms and a reduction in the number of sexual partners will greatly reduce, but not eliminate, the risk of infection. Oral exposure to semen and vaginal secretions has been implicated in transmission of HIV occasionally, and female-to-female transmission has been documented. HIV has been isolated from saliva, but at much lower concentration than is found in blood. There is no clear evidence of transmission via saliva. On the other hand, there is no definitive proof that prolonged, deep kissing cannot transmit HIV.

Sharing of Intravenous Needles: Sharing of needles, syringes, or other devices that allow parenteral introduction of infected blood, carries a high risk of HIV transmission.

Perinatal Transmission: The risk of an HIV-infected mother transmitting HIV infection to her infant at or before birth is between 25 and 40%. Breast feeding by postnatally infected mothers has also resulted in transmission of HIV to infants.

Occupational Transmission: The best available estimate of the risk of HIV infection following a single parenteral (needle-stick) exposure to HIV infected blood is 0.4%, or approximately one infection per 250 exposures. Exposed health care providers may choose to take prophylactic AZT (see below). In several studies of health care workers, HIV infection following a mucous membrane exposure (mouth or eye splash of blood or body fluids) has not occurred. It is reasonable to assume that the risk from a splash exposure is much less than the risk following a parenteral exposure.

Blood or Blood Product Transfusions: Since blood banks began testing blood for the presence of antibodies to HIV and taking protective measures in the mid-1980's, the risk of acquiring HIV from a blood transfusion in the U.S. has fallen to about 1 in 100,000 per unit, with estimates ranging from 1 in 40,000 to 1 in 225,000 (ref. 19). Approximately half of all hemophiliacs in the U.S. before 1984 were infected by transfusion of clotting factors infected with HIV.

Other Considerations: HIV is NOT transmitted by insect bites, by casual or household contact, or by contact with the sweat or intact skin of an infected person. Factor VIII and cryoprecipitate produced after 1984 are heat-treated to inactivate viruses, substantially reducing the risk of infection. Immune serum globulin, including RhoGam, does not transmit HIV, as the method of preparation inactivates viruses. Donating blood does not pose any risk of HIV infection to the donor.

III. Prevention

A) Risk Reduction: (3)

As there is no known cure for AIDS, prevention of infection is of paramount importance. The physician must educate patients about risk factors for HIV transmission, and assist patients in modifying high-risk behaviors. Judgmental attitudes on the part of physicians or staff may interfere with compassionate patient care. No matter what the route of potential transmission, patients should be informed that infectivity cannot be ruled out on the basis of appearance, state of health, or social standing.

Risk of sexual transmission is reduced by avoiding high-risk activities (especially anal and vaginal intercourse) with partners at high or unknown risk of HIV infection. Use of latex condoms with water-based lubricant, containing a virucidal agent (e.g., nonoxynol-9), during anal or vaginal penetration; use of condoms during fellatio; use of latex patches (dental dams) during cunnilingus; and avoidance of alcohol and drugs in amounts that impair judgement are practices which will reduce risk of transmission.

Experimentation with IV drugs by non-users should be discouraged, and every effort should be made to get established users into drug treatment programs. For those who are unwilling or unable to discontinue IV drugs, the importance of not sharing needles should be stressed. If needles are shared, the needle and syringe should be cleaned with a dilute bleach solution (1 part household bleach to 10 parts water), and then rinsed with clean water.

Women with or at high risk of HIV infection should be encouraged to avoid pregnancy. The HIV-infected woman who is already pregnant should receive counseling to enable her to make an informed decision about abortion. In industrialized countries, breast feeding is not essential to a child's health, and should be discouraged in HIV-infected women (4).

Persons at risk for HIV infection must not donate blood, even if their HIV antibody test is negative. False negatives can occur, especially in the first several months following exposure; blood donated by such patients may escape detection by blood banks. Transfusion therapy should be reserved for those patients with a compelling need for blood or blood products.

B) Prevention of Occupational HIV Transmission, Body Substance Precautions:

Needles should never be re-capped using both hands; if recapping is necessary, the cap should be placed on a flat surface, and the needle inserted into it. Sharp objects should be deposited into a puncture-proof disposal container as soon as possible.

Gloves should be worn whenever touching mucous membranes or broken skin, whenever there is a risk of contact with body fluids, and whenever any invasive procedure, including venipuncture, is performed. The amount of blood introduced, and the risk of infection by an accidental needle stick is reduced if the stick occurs through a glove. Gloves should also be worn to protect hand cuts, abrasions or rashes. Gowns should be worn when patient care is expected to soil clothing, as in the presence of active bleeding, incontinence or vomiting. Protective goggles and mask should be worn when splash or aerosol droplet exposure is likely. Protective clothing is unnecessary and inappropriate in the absence of exposure risks.

Hands and other skin surfaces exposed to blood or body fluids should be washed with soap and water, and mucous membranes should be flooded with water or saline.

C) Post-Exposure Prophylaxis: (5,6)

At San Francisco General Hospital, prophylactic treatment with zidovudine (AZT, Retrovir) is routinely encouraged for health care workers following significant occupational exposure to HIV. The efficacy of AZT in preventing infection with HIV following occupational exposure is not known, and treatment with AZT in this setting has failed to prevent seroconversion in a least three known cases (P. Volberding, personal communication). Based in part on animal experiments, it is presumed that post-exposure AZT may be effective in slowing the progression of HIV disease, whether or not infection is prevented.

Significant exposure is defined as contact, via percutaneous injury, mucous membrane or broken skin, with blood, body fluids, or tissue from an HIV infected patient. Transfusion and intramuscular injection carry a particularly high risk of seroconversion. If the HIV status of the source patient is unknown (or if the patient refuses testing), treatment may be started pending HIV testing, depending on the severity of exposure.

Workers with prior history of HIV infection, those who are pregnant or breast feeding, and those who have illnesses that contraindicate treatment with AZT are generally advised against post-exposure prophylaxis. Men and women receiving AZT should use contraception during the four weeks of treatment and during the subsequent four weeks because of the mutagenic potential of AZT.

Prophylaxis should be initiated as soon as possible, preferably within one hour, and no later than 72 hours following exposure (delays in treatment are associated with chemoprophylaxis failures in animal models). HIV antibody testing should be provided as soon as possible following exposure to document baseline serostatus. Follow-up testing is recommended at 6 weeks, 3 months, and 6 months.

Post-Exposure Prophylactic Treatment:
Zidovudine (AZT), 200 mg po q 4 hours (or 6 times a day) for the first 72

hours, followed by an additional 25 days at a dosage of either 200 mg po 5 times a day, or 100 mg 5 times a day. The side effects of AZT are discussed below.

IV. HIV Testing Methods & Natural History of HIV Infection: (7,8)

HIV Seroconversion and Testing Methods:

The development of detectable antibodies to HIV (seroconversion) usually occurs within 3 months of infection, but occasionally seroconversion occurs six months or longer after infection. Antibody testing usually consists of an enzyme-linked immunosorbent assay (ELISA), a highly sensitive screening test. If the result is positive, the ELISA is repeated, and if the repeat is also positive, a Western blot test, a highly specific test, is performed for confirmation.

Mechanisms of HIV Disease:

Because the HIV retroviral genome is integrated into the DNA of infected cells (including T-helper lymphocytes, B-lymphocytes, macrophages, brain glial cells, and Langerhans cells in the skin), infection with HIV persists throughout the lifetime of the infected individual, and will not be eradicated by antiviral therapy.

The derangement of immune function characteristic of AIDS is probably due, at least partially, to the loss of T-helper cells. The normal CD4 count in healthy, non-HIV infected individuals is approximately 1200 per microliter (cubic mm), while most serious opportunistic infections tend to occur at counts of 200 or fewer CD4 lymphocytes per microliter.

After infection with HIV, T-helper (CD4) lymphocyte counts decline with considerable variability from patient to patient at a rate of roughly 80-100 cells per microliter per year. The rate of decline may also vary at different stages in the course of the disease. Approximately 85% of patients with fewer than 200 CD4 cells per microliter will develop an AIDS-defining diagnosis within 3 years, and approximately half of individuals infected with HIV develop an AIDS-defining illness within 10 years of infection. (AIDS is diagnosed when an AIDS-defining opportunistic infection or malignancy occurs; see Clinical Category C, page 11.)

Manifestations of HIV Disease:

Acute HIV Infection (Seroconversion Illness):
A substantial portion of HIV-infected persons develop a mononucleosis-like syndrome (primary HIV infection, seroconversion illness) 2 to 4 weeks after being infected. Symptoms last several days to several weeks, and may include fever, sore throat, malaise, and sometimes a measles-like rash.

Asymptomatic Phase:
HIV infection may remain asymptomatic for many years following sero-conversion. Enlargement of peripheral lymph nodes may occur, and

commonly persists for months or years following seroconversion.

In addition to the AIDS-defining illnesses (Category C, below), the following conditions are more common or more severe, or both, in the setting of HIV infection.

Constitutional Disease:
As HIV disease progresses, patients may develop constitutional symptoms, including weight loss, chronic fevers, myalgias, and night sweats. Megestrol acetate (Megace), 80 mg po tid-qid, may increase appetite and result in weight gain in patients with anorexia and weight loss. Impotence is a common side effect of doses exceeding 300 mg per day.
Neurologic and Psychiatric Diseases:
Cerebrovascular events (transient ischemic attacks or stroke), vacuolar myelopathy, and peripheral neuropathies all occur in HIV infection. HIV encephalopathy (AIDS dementia complex) is diagnostic of AIDS, and usually occurs at CD4 levels below 200 per cu mm.
Affective disorders are common in HIV infection; depression may cause signs mimicking early encephalopathy (attention, concentration, or memory deficits; psychomotor slowing, apathy or agitation) at any stage of illness. Mania is also observed.
Secondary Infectious Diseases:
HIV infection is associated with greater frequency and/or severity of bacterial pneumonias (often due to S. pneumoniae, H. influenzae, Staph, Branhamella, or gram-negative rods), bacterial sepsis, chronic sinusitis (refs. 24,25), pulmonary tuberculosis, syphilis, pelvic inflammatory disease, salmonellosis (raw eggs should be avoided) listeriosis (unpasteurized dairy products should be avoided), nocardiosis, bacillary angiomatosis, herpes simplex, herpes zoster, candidiasis, extra-intestinal strongyloidiasis, oral hairy leukoplakia.
Neoplasms:
Kaposi's sarcoma (KS), while technically diagnostic of AIDS, may occur earlier in the course of HIV disease than other AIDS-defining opportunistic infections. Diagnosis of KS should be made by skin biopsy, since other conditions (bacillary angiomatosis, which responds to erythromycin) may cause skin lesions of similar appearance.
The rate of cervical intraepithelial neoplasia in women and anal intraepithelial neoplasia in men is increased in the setting of HIV infection. Cervical cancer may occur at T-cell levels higher than usually associated with the diagnosis of AIDS, although the frequency and severity of cervical neoplasia increases as CD4 counts decrease. The risk of anal cancer also appears to increase with increasing immunosuppression.
HIV-associated Non-Hodgkin lymphoma (see ref. 20 for a review), although diagnostic of AIDS, may present at variable levels of immune function, with survival directly related to level of immune competence.

While >90% of AIDS-associated lymphomas are of the non-Hodgkin type, the incidence of Hodgkin disease (not considered diagnostic of AIDS) is also increased in the setting of HIV infection (21).

Hematologic Disorders:
Conditions occurring in HIV infected patients, often before the diagnosis of an AIDS-defining condition, include anemia (see ref. 22 for review), leuko penias, immune thrombocytopenia (ITP), and thrombotic thrombocytopenic purpura (TTP) (ref. 23).

Dermatologic conditions (9):
Folliculitis, seborrheic dermatitis, dry skin, dermatophytosis, and molluscum contagiosum are common in HIV infection. Cutaneous manifestations are also associated with several opportunistic infections, including pneumocystosis, histoplasmosis, coccidioidomycosis (papular rashes), tuberculosis (abscesses), and Herpesviruses (vesicles). Kaposi's sarcoma and bacillary angiomatosis usually manifest as purplish skin lesions.

Other conditions: Myopathy, nephropathy often characterized by severe nephrotic syndrome (26), myocarditis, cardiomyopathy, Reiter's syndrome, adrenal insufficiency, gonadal insufficiency, and pituitary insufficiency are all observed in HIV infection without established etiology.

Revised Centers for Disease Control (CDC) HIV Classification System and Expanded AIDS Surveillance Definition for Adolescents and Adults (unadopted as of September 1992):

The revised system utilizes the CD4 lymphocyte count to classify HIV infected patients. The system is based on three clinical categories and three CD4 ranges. Individual patients are classified based on a matrix using the CD4 count and three categories. To classify a given patient, determine the clinical category, then match with the CD4 count on the matrix. Nine exclusive categories are possible.

 3 months); acute HIV illness.

Clinical Category B:*
    Bacterial endocarditis, meningitis, pneumonia, sepsis.
    Candidiasis, vulvovaginal; more than 1 month duration
    Candidiasis, oropharyngeal.
    Cervical dysplasia, severe or carcinoma.
    Constitutional symptoms such as fever >38.5°, or prolonged diarrhea >1
        month.
    Hairy leukoplakia, oral.
    Herpes zoster, ≥ 2 episodes or > 1 dermatome
    Idiopathic thrombocytopenic purpura.
    Listeriosis
    M. tuberculosis, pulmonary
    Nocardiosis
    Pelvic inflammatory disease

Peripheral neuropathy.

* These illnesses must be attributable to HIV infection or have a clinical course complicated by HIV disease.

Clinical Category C (Consists of AIDS-defining illnesses by the 1987 CDC definition (ref. 2) currently in use):

Candidiasis: esophageal, tracheal, bronchial.

Coccidiomycosis, extrapulmonary.

Cryptococcosis, extrapulmonary.

Cryptosporidiosis, chronic intestinal, with diarrhea lasting > 1 month.

Cytomegalovirus retinitis or disease of other than liver, spleen, lymph nodes.

HIV encephalopathy ("AIDS dementia complex").

Herpes simplex with mucocutaneous ulcer > 1 month duration; or causing bronchitis, pneumonia, or esophagitis.

Histoplasmosis (disseminated).

Isosporiasis, with diarrhea lasting > 1 month.

Kaposi's sarcoma.

Non-Hodgkin Lymphoma: Burkitt's (small non-cleaved), immunoblastic sarcoma, or primary CNS lymphoma.

M. avium or M. kansasii, extrapulmonary

M. tuberculosis, extrapulmonary

Mycobacterium, other species disseminated or extrapulmonary.

Pneumocystis carinii pneumonia.

Progressive multifocal leukoencephalopathy.

Salmonella bacteremia, recurrent.

Toxoplasmosis, cerebral.

Wasting syndrome due to HIV.

Classification System Matrix

	Clinical Category		
CD4 cell count	A	B	C
(1) ≥ 500/mm3	A1	B1	C1
(2) 200-499	A2	B2	C2
(3) < 200	A3	B3	C3

AIDS Surveillance Definition: Shaded areas indicate expanded CDC clinical definition of AIDS.

Note: Due to diurnal variation in CD4 levels, blood samples for sequential CD4 levels should be drawn at same time of day each time.

V. Clinical evaluation of the HIV-infected patient (10)

A) History and physical exam should address the signs and symptoms of HIV infection described above, as well as those of specific opportunistic infections.

Pertinent History in Patients with HIV Infection:
-Level of progression of HIV disease, by length of infection or prior CD4 counts.
-History of comorbid infections including tuberculosis, syphilis, herpes simplex, and herpes zoster; and treatment received.
-Travel to or residence in areas endemic for coccidioidomycosis (Southwestern US, San Joaquin Valley, Northern Mexico), histoplasmosis (Mississippi & Ohio River valleys, Caribbean), tuberculosis (Southeast Asia, homeless shelters or IV drug-using communities in urban US), or other infections.
-Prior positive PPD or known TB exposure.
-Medications and possible drug reactions.

Symptoms:
Systemic: Decreased energy level, anorexia, weight loss, fevers, night sweats.
Skin: Rashes, itching, dryness, pigmented lesions.
Lymphatics: Increase or decrease in size of lymph nodes.
HEENT: Headache, visual changes, sinus congestion, oral lesions.
Cardiopulmonary: Cough, dyspnea, chest pain.
Gastrointestinal: Dysphagia, odynophagia, abdominal pain, nausea, vomiting, diarrhea.
Musculoskeletal: Myalgias, arthralgias.
Neuro/psych: speech changes, memory loss, neuralgias, weakness, confusion, depression, neck stiffness.

Physical Exam Findings:
Skin: Seborrhea, folliculitis, Kaposi's sarcoma lesions (purplish-brown pigmented macules), psoriasis, fungal lesions, herpetic lesions, molluscum papules.
Lymphatics: Asymmetric or tender lymph nodes.
Eyes: Visual acuity and fields, fundal exudates or hemorrhages.
Mouth: Hairy leukoplakia, thrush, aphthous ulcers, Kaposi's sarcoma.
Cardiopulmonary: Murmur in intravenous drug users, focal lung findings.
Gastrointestinal: hepatosplenomegaly.
Pelvic: Candidiasis, condyloma, Pap smear.
Rectal: Perianal lesions (herpes vs. gonorrhea), condyloma, fissures, proctitis, anal masses (consider anal Pap smear or biopsy of lesion if condyloma or mass present).
Neuro/psych: Motor, sensory, and mental status exams.

B) Initial Laboratory Evaluation of HIV-infected Patients:

-CBC with differential and platelets.
-Baseline electrolytes, BUN, creatinine, and liver function tests.
-CD4 count, for staging disease and determining when to initiate Pneumocystis carinii pneumonia prophylaxis and anti-retroviral therapy (see below).
-Lactate dehydrogenase (LDH) baseline level (increases suggest PCP or lymphoma).
-Glucose-6-phosphate dehydrogenase (G6PD) level, especially in dark-skinned patients, to assess safety of potential treatment with dapsone or primaquine (see chapter on PCP).
-Hepatitis B serologies (surface antigen and anti-surface antibody).
-Syphilis screening (VDRL or RPR) (see chapter on syphilis).
-PPD tuberculin test with controls (see chapter on tuberculosis).
-Some physicians favor a baseline chest X-ray.

VI. Health Maintenance

A) Periodic Reassessment: Following initial evaluation, the following tests should be performed regularly in patients with HIV infection:

1) CD4 counts every 3-6 months. Counts may vary between laboratories, may be lowered by concomitant viral infections, and may show diurnal variation (higher in morning). The trend is more reliable than any single count.
2) Purified protein derivative for tuberculosis (PPD) with controls q 12 months, until patient becomes **anergic**.
3) VDRL or RPR for syphilis q 12 months if patient is sexually active.
4) Pap smear q 6 months in women.
5) Serum cryptococcal antigen (CrAg) should be monitored frequently in patients with CD4 counts <100.

B) Preventive Care: Unless contraindicated, HIV-infected patients should receive:
1) Pneumococcal vaccine
2) Hepatitis B vaccine (if HBsAb negative and at risk)
3) Influenza vaccine (in season)
The earlier in the course of HIV infection a vaccine is given, the more likely patients are to respond. Live vaccines, such as yellow fever, oral polio, and BCG should be avoided.

C) Pneumocystis Carinii Pneumonia Prophylaxis:
HIV-infected patients with fewer than 200 CD4 cells per microliter (and probably those with somewhat higher CD4 counts and severe constitutional

symptoms, thrush, or hairy leukoplakia) should be started on prophylaxis against pneumocystis carinii pneumonia (PCP). (See chapter on PCP for regimens.) The utility of prophylaxis against other opportunistic infections (cryptococcus, toxoplasma, Mycobacterium avium complex) is under investigation.

D) Anti-HIV Therapy: (11,12,13)

1) Zidovudine (Retrovir, azidothymidine, AZT), HIV-infected patients with fewer than 500 CD4 cells per microliter should begin anti-retroviral chemotherapy with zidovudine (AZT). Many authorities believe that patients with rapidly falling CD4 counts (i.e., loss of >100-150 cells per microliter per year) should also be started on antiviral therapy. This nucleoside analog has been shown, based on randomized, placebo controlled trials, to prolong survival and decrease the frequency of opportunistic infections in patients with advanced HIV infection (14). AZT has also been shown to decrease progression to AIDS in asymptomatic and mildly symptomatic HIV-infected persons with CD4 counts below 500 cells per microliter (15,16). The value of AZT in HIV-infected individuals with CD4 counts above 500 is under investigation.

Zidovudine (AZT) Dosage: in both asymptomatic and symptomatic patients with CD4 counts under 500, or with rapidly falling CD4 counts:
Zidovudine (AZT), 200 mg po tid, or 500 mg po per day, divided into 3 doses per day (i.e., 200-100-200). This dosage appears to provide an optimum balance between efficacy and toxicity (11). Dosages as low as 300 mg per day may have anti-HIV activity, but should probably be reserved for patients with drug toxicity.

Dose-limiting side effects of AZT:

Macrocytic anemia (unresponsive to vitamin B12), sometimes severe.
Neutropenia
Thrombocytopenia
Toxic myopathy (after long-term treatment with AZT)
Hepatitis (infrequent).

Initial side effects of AZT: weakness, headache, dizziness, sleep disturbances, anorexia, nausea, vomiting, malaise, and myalgias. These symptoms usually diminish over several weeks with continued use, and seldom require lowering dosage or discontinuation of the drug. Serious side effects are less frequent in asymptomatic patients taking AZT than in patients with advanced HIV disease.

Management of Zidovudine (AZT) Therapy:

-Monitor CBC with differential and platelets every two weeks for the first month of treatment, and every 1 to 3 months thereafter. Close monitoring for myelotoxicity is necessary when combining AZT with other myelosuppressive drugs, such as ganciclovir, TMP-SMX, or antineoplastic chemotherapeutic agents; many clinicians interrupt AZT therapy during induction therapy with myelosuppressive drugs. AZT should probably not be used in any patient with a hemoglobin of less than 7.5 mg/dl or absolute neutrophil count less than 750 cells/microliter.

-Anemia may be managed with transfusion, with erythropoietin, or by changing to a non-myelosuppressive antiviral (see below). Colony stimulating factors (GM-CSF or G-CSF) may increase neutrophil counts in AZT-induced neutropenia. The use of non- myelotoxic drugs for opportunistic infections (e.g., foscarnet instead of ganciclovir for CMV retinitis) may facilitate concomitant use of AZT.

-Monitor liver function tests and CPK every 3 months.

-Avoid probenecid, which prolongs the serum half-life of AZT.

-Strains of HIV with in-vitro resistance to AZT may emerge within the first six to twelve months of treatment with AZT in patients with advanced HIV disease. Appearance of resistant viruses takes much longer in asymptomatic patients treated with AZT. The clinical significance of in-vitro resistance is not clear. AZT-resistant isolates are susceptible in vitro to ddI and ddC, suggesting a role for combination therapy, but there is little data available to support any given regimen. It is not known, for example, whether a patient started on ddI, because of progression of disease while on AZT, should also continue to receive AZT to suppress AZT-susceptible strains.

For a review of the role of AZT, see reference 27.

2) Didanosine (ddI): The nucleoside analog dideoxyinosine (ddI, didanosine, Videx) has been shown in uncontrolled trials to increase CD4 counts and reduce viral antigenemia in patients with advanced HIV infection. The drug is approved for use in patients intolerant to, or deteriorating despite, treatment with AZT. Studies directly comparing ddI to AZT are pending.

Dose of Didanosine by Body Weight:

Weight (kg)	Dose (po)
≥75	300 mg bid
50-74	200 mg bid
35-49	125 mg bid

Serious side effects of ddI include peripheral neuropathy (primarily sensory) and pancreatitis; each of these effects occurs with a rate of 5-20% after 12 months of treatment. The risk of pancreatitis, which may be fatal, is increased in patients with a history of pancreatitis or exposure to pentamidine. Neuropathy is reversible if it is recognized promptly and ddI is rapidly discontinued. Diarrhea, due to the alkaline buffer with which ddI is administered, is common. Confusion, rash, leukopenia, and elevated transaminase levels have also occurred.

DDI is destroyed by gastric acid, and should not be taken with food. Each dose of ddI must be given as at least two tablets adding up to the desired dose, as no single tablet contains adequate buffer to provide the high pH necessary for absorption. Tablets must be crushed or chewed before swallowing. Drugs requiring low gastric pH for absorption (such as dapsone and ketoconazole) should not be taken within two hours of ddI, as the buffer prevents their absorption. Patients taking ddI should receive frequent neurologic sensory exams, and should be instructed to report any distal pain or numbness. Serum amylase should be followed, as an increase may precede pancreatitis.

3) Dideoxycytidine (ddC):

The nucleoside analog dideoxycytidine (ddC, zalcitabine, Hivid) has been used to treat advanced HIV infection alone and in combination with AZT (18). ddC was approved by the FDA in mid-1992 for use, in combination with AZT, in adult HIV patients with CD4 count <300 and clinical or immunological deterioration on AZT alone.

The optimum dose of ddC is unclear. The manufacturer's recommended dose of ddC is 0.75 mg po tid, given in combination with AZT, 600 mg per day. Some physicians prefer to use 0.375 mg tid with AZT. Used alone, ddC appears to be less active than AZT; ddI is probably preferable to ddC for single-agent therapy in patients intolerant or resistant to AZT (P.A. Volberding, personal communication, 1992).

The major toxic side effects of ddC are peripheral neuropathy and pancreatitis, both of which may occur less frequently with ddC than with ddI. Other side effects include elevation in LFT's, rash, fever, and aphthous stomatitis during the first month of treatment, as well as esophageal ulcerations. Patients taking ddC should receive frequent neurological exams and monitoring of serum amylase (as with ddI; see above) as well as LFT's.

4) Combination and Alternation Therapy

There is good evidence that the combination of AZT plus ddI, like the combination of AZT plus ddC, is more active against HIV than AZT alone. There is a lack of consensus, however, as to whether combination therapy should be instituted at the outset of treatment, or reserved for patients progressing (new opportunistic infections, rapidly falling CD4 counts) despite AZT therapy.

Authorities at SFGH recommend combination therapy for any patient initially presenting with a CD4 count of <200, or presenting with an opportunistic infection at any CD4 count, as well as for patients with progressive disease on AZT alone (J.D. Stansell, personal communication, 1992). When combination therapy is used, each drug should be given at full dose, as toxicities of ddI and ddC do not overlap with those of AZT.

One study (17) has shown that patients with AZT-resistant HIV regained sensitivity to AZT after being switched to ddI for approximately one year. Analysis suggests that mutations associated with ddI resistance change the structure of the viral reverse transcriptase in such a way that AZT resistance is lost. This study suggests a role for concurrent administration of both ddI and AZT, or for switching back and forth between the two drugs at, for example, monthly intervals.

A recently published study (28) showed a reduction in the incidence of new opportunistic infections when ddI, 500 mg/d, was given to patients who had already received long-term (median 14 months) AZT therapy. This benefit was seen in patients with low CD4 counts who were asymptomatic or mildly symptomatic, but not in those with AIDS diagnoses. No effect on survival was found.

5) Investigational Drug: d4T

The nucleoside analog d4T (stavudine) compares favorably with AZT, ddI, and ddC in efficacy and toxicity according to early studies (29), and is available through an expanded access program (Bristol-Meyers-Squibb, 1-800-842-8036) free of charge for patients failing or intolerant to both AZT and ddI.

References

1) Centers for Disease Control. The Second 100,000 cases of Acquired Immunodeficiency Syndrome -- United States, June 1981 - December 1991. MMWR 1992; 41:28-29.
2) Centers for Disease Control. Revision of the CDC Surveillance Case Definition for Acquired Immunodeficiency Syndrome. MMWR 1987; 26:3S-15S.
3) Wofsy CB. Prevention of HIV Transmission. In Sande MA and Volberding PA, eds. Medical Management of AIDS, 2nd ed. 1990. Saunders; Philadelphia: 38-56.
4) Stiehm ER and FP Vinck. Transmission of Human Immunodeficiency Virus Infection by Breast Feeding. Journal of Pediatrics 1991; 118:410-412.
5) Beckman SE, et al. Risky Business: Using necessarily imprecise casualty counts to estimate occupational risks for HIV-1 Infection. Infec Control Hosp Epidemiol 1991; 11:371-379.
6) Henderson DK and JL Gerberding. Prophylactic zidovudine after occupational exposure to the Human Immunodeficiency Virus Type 1: An Interim Analysis. Journal of Infectious Diseases 1989; 160:321-327.
7) Kiefer RG and SB Hulley. Understanding the AIDS Epidemic: I. Emergence of the Epidemic and Natural History of the Disease. In Petrow, s, et al., eds.

Ending the HIV Epidemic: Community Strategies in Disease Prevention and Health Promotion. ETR Network Publications; Santa Cruz. 1990.

8) Northfelt DW, ed. "Focus on HIV Malignancies." AIDSFILE 1992; 6:1-10. (Contributions by Northfelt on Kaposi's sarcoma, L. Kaplan on lymphoma, M. Maiman on cervical cancer, and J. Palefsky on anal cancer.)

9) Berger TG, et al. Dermatologic Manifestations of HIV infection. American Family Physician 1990; 41:1729-1742.

10) Hollander H and MH Katz. AIDS and Related Conditions. In Current Medical Diagnosis and Treatment 1991. Schroeder SA, et al., eds. Appleton and Lange; San Mateo: 939-951.

11) Volberding PA. Update on Nucleosides. AIDSFILE 1991; 5:1-2.

12) Northfelt DW. Combination Antiretroviral Therapy for HIV Infection. AIDSFILE 1991; 5:5-7.

13) The Medical Letter on Drugs and Therapeutics. Drugs For Viral Infections. 1992; 34:31-36.

14) Fischl MA, et al. The Efficacy of AZT in the treatment of patients with AIDS and AIDS-Related Complex. NEJM 1987; 317:185-191.

15) Volberding PA, et al. Zidovudine in asymptomatic HIV infection. NEJM 1990; 322:941-949.

16) Hamilton JD et al. A Controlled Trial of Early vs. Late treatment with AZT in Symptomatic HIV Infection. Results of the Veterans Affairs Cooperative Study. NEJM 1992; 326:437-443.

17) St Clair MH, et al. Resistance to ddI and Sensitivity to AZT induced by a mutation in HIV-1 reverse Transcriptase. Science 1991; 253:1557-1559.

18) Meng TC, et al. Combination therapy with zidovudine and dideoxycytidine in patients with advanced HIV infections. A Phase I/II Study. Annals of Internal Medicine 1992;116:13-20.

19) Dodd RY. The risk of transfusion-transmitted infection. NEJM 1992; 327:419-421.

20) Levine AM. AIDS-related lymphoma. Blood 1992; 80:8-20.

21) Hessol NA, et al. Increased incidence of Hodgkin disease in homosexual men with HIV infection. Annals of Internal Medicine 1992; 117:309-311.

22) Doukas MA. HIV-associated anemia. Medical Clinics of North America 1992; 76:699-709.

23) Rarick MU, et al. Thrombotic thrombocytopenic purpura in patients with human immunodeficiency virus infection: a report of three cases and a review of the literature. American Journal of Hematology 1992; 40:103-9.

24) Godofsky, EW et al. Sinusitis in HIV-1 infected patients: a clinical and radiographic review. Am. J. Med. 1992; 93:163-70.

25) Zurlo JJ, et al. Sinusitis in HIV-1 infection. Am. J. Med. 1992; 93:157-62.

26) Burgoigne JJ and V Pardo. HIV-associated nephropathies. NEJM 1992; 327:729-30.

27) McLeod, GX and SM Hammer. Zidovudine: five years later. Annals of Internal Medicine 1992; 177:487-501.

28) Kahn JO, et al. A controlled trial comparing continued zidovudine with

dideoxyinosine in HIV infection. NEJM 1992; 327:581-587.
29) Dunkle L, et al. Stavudine (d4T): a promising antiretroviral agent. Abstract WeB 1011, VIII International Conference on AIDS, Amsterdam 1992.

Pneumocystis carinii

1. Introduction

Pneumocystis carinii pneumonia (PCP) is the most common AIDS-defining opportunistic infection in industrialized countries. Without prophylaxis, 80-85% of AIDS patients will develop PCP at some point. PCP has been the first AIDS-defining disease to occur in half of AIDS patients in the US, and has been the cause of death in about 25% of AIDS patients.

Rarely, pneumocystis can cause a disseminated infection involving the lymph nodes, spleen, liver and bone marrow, and, occasionally, the adrenals, thyroid, middle ear, or skin.

2. Presentation

History: Patients typically experience a prodrome lasting several weeks, consisting of low-grade fevers, drenching night sweats, weakness, and malaise. As the disease progresses, cough (non-productive or productive of white, frothy sputum) and dyspnea on exertion develop. While PCP alone does not cause purulent sputum, concomitant sinusitis is not uncommon. Therefore, the presence of purulent sputum does not by itself rule out PCP.

90% of patients with PCP have T-helper (CD4) count of <200 cells/microliter. Fewer than 1% of HIV-infected patients with CD_4 counts >500 will develop PCP.

Physical Exam: Non-specific. Fever, tachypnea, and tachycardia are common. Breath sounds are often decreased at lung bases, and deep inspiration usually elicits cough. In severe disease, crackles may be heard and cyanosis may be present.

Labs:

Arterial blood gas: Hypoxemia, sometimes acute respiratory alkalosis

LDH: Elevated by >50 IU from baseline in 90%.
-Mean serum LDH in PCP is 360 IU, as opposed to 224 in HIV patients with other causes of pulmonary disease (8).
-Differential diagnosis of elevated LDH includes acute myocardial infarction, hepatitis, pulmonary embolism, lymphoma, hemolysis, B12 or folate deficiency, muscle injury, renal infarct.

ESR: Sedimentation rate usually elevated.

Chest X-ray is variable (1,9):

The classic appearance is a diffuse perihilar and/or bibasilar, interstitial or reticulonodular, heterogeneous density. If untreated, infiltrates may progress within a few days to diffuse air space consolidation involving the entire lung.

Frequent variations include unilateral or focal heterogeneous infiltrates, apical infiltrates (typical of failed prophylaxis with aerosolized pentamidine), or pneumatoceles (bullae), which are found in 10% of patients. Pneumothorax develops in 2-9% of patients with PCP, while AIDS patients without PCP are not at an increased risk of pneumothorax (4,5).

Rarely a miliary pattern, focal alveolar consolidation or cavitary nodules occur. Pleural effusion due to PCP is very rare, and another cause of the effusion should be considered. The chest X-ray is <u>normal</u> in 5-10% of affected patients.

Differential diagnosis of pulmonary symptoms and signs (9,14,15):

The differential diagnosis of pulmonary symptoms in the HIV-positive patient includes bacterial pathogens (pneumococcus, hemophilus influenzae, and others), mycobacteria (tuberculosis and, less commonly, Mycobacterium avium complex), fungi (coccidioides, histoplasma, cryptococcus, and, rarely, nocardia, aspergillus, or candida), PCP, parasitic infection (toxoplasma or cryptosporidium, both rare), cytomegalovirus (rare), and non-infectious or idiopathic causes, including Kaposi's sarcoma, pulmonary lymphoma, and lymphocytic interstitial pneumonia (LIP), which is most common in children with AIDS.

<u>Bacterial pneumonias</u> are most often due to pneumococcus or hemophilus influenzae; staphylococcus and branhamella are also common. Bacterial pneumonias occur more frequently in HIV-positive patients than in seronegative controls, but with similar presentations (11). Symptoms include abrupt onset of fever, productive cough, dyspnea, and pleuritic chest pain. Localizing findings (rales, dullness to percussion, bronchial breath sounds, egophony) are frequently present on exam; a relative leukocytosis and left shift are usually present, and the chest X-ray is almost always abnormal, usually showing lobar or segmental consolidation, although diffuse infiltrates are common in hemophilus. Sputum usually contains neutrophils, and sputum culture is usually positive. Blood cultures are positive in 40-80% of HIV-positive patients with bacterial pneumonia.

The remaining entities are not distinguishable from each other or from PCP on imaging studies, and the clinician is obliged to pursue a series of diagnostic procedures as described in the next section.

There are few, if any, pathognomonic findings on chest X-ray in AIDS. When the patient's condition requires rapid institution of empirical therapy, however, the chest x-ray may be helpful (see table).

Radiographic Presentations of Pulmonary Diseases in HIV Patients:

Diffuse Interstitial/Alveolar Infiltrates
Pneumocystis
Kaposi's sarcoma
Cytomegalovirus (very rare)
Hemophilus influenzae
Toxoplasmosis (rare cause)
Disseminated Tuberculosis
Disseminated fungal infections

Reticulonodular/Micronodular Infiltrates
Tuberculosis (late in HIV disease)
Mycobacterium avium complex
Histoplasmosis
Coccidioides
PCP
Kaposi's sarcoma
Lymphocytic interstitial pneumonia

Focal Infiltrates
Bacterial pneumonias
PCP
TB (early in HIV disease)
Fungal infections (nodular)
MAC (very rare cause)
Septic emboli
Kaposi's sarcoma

Pleural Effusion
Kaposi's sarcoma
Lymphoma
Tuberculosis
Cryptococcus
Nocardia
Bacterial pneumonias

Intrathoracic Adenopathy
TB (late in HIV disease)
10% of Kaposi's sarcoma
6-20% of Mycobacterium avium
25% of lymphoma
Histo, cocci (unusual)
cryptococcus
Not HIV-associated
  lymphadenopathy

Cavity
TB
Aspergillus
Nocardia
Cryptococcus
Staph aureus
PCP (pneumatocele)
Coccidioides (unusual)

3. Diagnostic algorithm for Pneumocystis carinii pneumonia:

Definitive diagnosis of PCP consists in detection of the organism in respiratory secretions. At San Francisco General Hospital (SFGH), the following sequence is used in the diagnosis of an HIV-positive (or suspected HIV-positive) patient with respiratory symptoms as described above:

```
       Screening                                        Diagnostic
              abnormal, consistent with PCP*
Chest X-ray --------------------------------> |
 |  (normal)                                   |
 V                            <75% exp. |              negative      negative
Diffusing capacity CO** --------------> |-------->Sputum -------->BAL------>TBB
 |  (normal)                                   |      Induction
 V                  3 - 4+                     |
Gallium Scan ----------------------------> |
 | 0-2+
 V
Observe
```

Note: BAL - bronchoalveolar lavage; TBB - transbronchial biopsy

Each of the three screening tests (chest x-ray, diffusing capacity of carbon monoxide, pulmonary gallium scan) has an independent sensitivity of approximately 90% at SFGH, but is nonspecific (<50%) (ref. 10). Therefore, if any of the three is positive, the next logical step is to proceed to sputum induction. If all three are negative, the probability of PCP is low, and the patient may be observed without further work-up. Note: All coughing patients with abnormal chest x-rays should be placed in respiratory isolation until a diagnosis of PCP is established or tuberculosis has been ruled out.

Sputum induction is 70-80% sensitive at SFGH; therefore, a negative result necessitates bronchoscopy with broncho-alveolar lavage (BAL), which is 96-99% sensitive. BAL and transbronchial biopsy (TBB) taken together are virtually 100% sensitive for PCP at SFGH, so that TBB should be performed if there is strong clinical suspicion of PCP but BAL is negative. Because of the attendant risk of pneumothorax (about 9%), TBB is not done initially when PCP alone is suspected.

All three diagnostic procedures are highly specific; however, pneumocystis organisms are detectable in sputum and bronchial washings for at least 6 weeks following successful treatment of PCP, and do not necessarily signify active disease in this setting.

 * Patients with a chest X-ray and clinical presentation consistent with

bacterial pneumonia are treated with antibiotics, and sputum induction is not performed.

** Note that DLCO will generally be subnormal, and therefore not useful in diagnosing PCP, in the following settings:
   1) Prior pulmonary disease, including PCP
   2) Known pulmonary fibrosis
   3) Emphysema
   4) Talc granulomatosis in intravenous drug users

Prior to each of the diagnostic procedures, including sputum induction, the patient must take nothing by mouth for 8 hours. (Retching is common during sputum induction, and gastric contents render a sputum sample unusable.)

4. Treatment of Pneumocystis carinii Pneumonia:

Given a clinical impression of probable PCP, anti-PCP therapy should not be delayed pending diagnostic tests. Prompt treatment will in no way jeopardize subsequent diagnosis. A full course of therapy for PCP consists of 21 days of any one, or serial combination, of the following regimens:

a) Trimethoprim / Sulfamethoxazole Therapy, Treatment of Choice:

1) Trimethoprim/Sulfamethoxazole (Septra, Co-trimoxazole, TMP/SMX), 15 mg TMP/kg body weight/day, IV, divided into 3 or 4 doses per day, is the antibiotic of choice in severe PCP.

2) In mild to moderate disease ($PaO_2 > 70$ mmHg in room air), TMP/SMX, 2 double-strength tablets (each DS tablet contains 160 mg TMP/800 mg SMX), po tid to qid.

TMP/SMX is contraindicated in patients with sulfa allergy, as evidenced by Stevens-Johnson syndrome, exfoliative dermatitis, or anaphylaxis. Adverse reaction to TMP/SMX occurs in up to 60% of HIV-infected patients who receive the drug. Most frequently, reaction consists of a maculopapular rash that does not involve the mucous membranes, often associated with fever. Subsequent re-challenge with TMP/SMX may rarely cause a severe allergic reaction. If alternative therapies are not available, re-challenge with TMP/SMX may be attempted with close monitoring and follow-up of the patient.

Side Effects of TMP/SMX:

Nausea and vomiting. Usually worse when IV drug exceeds 350-400 mg TMP per dose. May be improved by giving smaller doses four times a day. May be treated symptomatically with lorazepam (Ativan), prochlorperazine (Compazine), or metoclopramide (Reglan).

<u>Fever</u>. Usually precedes appearance of rash. Fever and rash occur 7-10 days after beginning therapy with TMP/SMX. May be treated with acetaminophen or ibuprofen.

<u>Rash</u>. If mild and without blistering or mucous membrane involvement, may treat with antihistamines/antipruritics (e.g., diphenhydramine (benadryl), 50 mg q 6 hrs, or hydroxyzine (Atarax), 25 mg po q 6 hrs, plus Doxepin, 25 mg po qhs), and monitor closely for progression.

<u>Myelosuppression</u>: neutropenia (common), thrombocytopenia, anemia

<u>Hepatitis</u>.

Management of TMP/SMX Therapy:

-Monitor CBC, absolute neutrophil count (ANC), platelets, liver function tests.

-Do not give folate supplements. Folate negates the antibiotic effect of TMP.

-Infiltrates may appear worse on chest X-ray within first few days of treatment. Gas exchange may also worsen in the first 2-5 days of treatment, probably as a result of acute inflammatory reaction initiated by the killing of pneumocystis organisms. The large volume of fluid associated with IV TMP/SMX may also contribute to the worsening of gas exchange.

-In hyponatremic patients, give TMP/SMX in the minimum possible volume. If desired, drug may be given in NS instead of the usual D5W, but infusion must begin immediately after mixing, as the stability of TMP/SMX in saline is unknown.

b) <u>Alternative PCP Treatments:</u>

1) Primaquine/Clindamycin Therapy:

The combination of primaquine base, 30 mg po qd, plus clindamycin, 450-600 mg tid po or IV, is effective in patients unable to tolerate TMP/SMX. Side effects are generally less significant than those of pentamidine.

Each 26.4 mg tablet of primaquine contains 15 mg of the base form. The daily dose is therefore two 26.4 mg tablets.

Side Effects of Primaquine/Clindamycin:

Primaquine:
    <u>Hemolytic anemia</u> in G6PD deficiency
    <u>Methemoglobinemia</u>
    <u>Neutropenia</u> (usually less severe than with trimethoprim)
    <u>Leukocytosis</u>
    <u>Nausea and vomiting</u>

Headache
Clindamycin:
Nausea, vomiting, diarrhea
Pseudomembranous colitis
Combination:
The majority of patients on primaquine/clindamycin will develop a pruritic rash on day 8 - 12 of treatment. Treat symptomatically with antihistamines and antipruritics (eg, diphenhydramine (Benadryl), 50 mg q 6 hrs, or hydroxyzine (Atarax), 25 mg po q 6 hrs, plus doxepin, 25 mg po qhs).

Before treating with primaquine/clindamycin, check G6PD level. During treatment, suspect methemoglobinemia as with dapsone (See above).

2) Pentamidine Therapy:
In patients with severe PCP who fail to improve with, or are unable to tolerate, TMP/SMX, pentamidine may be used. The dose is:

Pentamidine isethionate, 3-4 mg/kg/d IV as a single daily dose, infused over at least 1 hr.

Side Effects of Pentamidine Therapy:

Hypotension
Arrhythmias (Ventricular tachycardia)
Hypoglycemia, usually after first 5-7 days of treatment
Hyperglycemia may occur up to months after treatment, in about 5% of patients with a history of hypoglycemia.
Hyperkalemia
Hypocalcemia
Hypomagnesemia
Myelotoxicity: neutropenia, pancytopenia
Nephrotoxicity, possibly progressing to acute renal failure
Acute pancreatitis
Elevated liver enzymes.

Management of Pentamidine Therapy:

-Monitor daily glucose, BUN, creatinine; frequent lytes, CBC with differential, platelets, calcium, liver function tests.
-If serum creatinine rises to 2.0-2.5 mg/dl, pentamidine should be discontinued. The drug may be restarted when creatinine is less than or equal to 1.5 mg/dl.
-Assure adequate fluid status before administering pentamidine.
-Avoid other nephrotoxic drugs (amphotericin B, aminoglycosides, vancomycin) whenever possible.

3) Trimethoprim/Dapsone Therapy:

The combination of trimethoprim, 15 mg/kg/d po in four divided doses, plus dapsone, 100 mg po qd, is equally effective as oral TMP/SMX in mild to moderate cases of PCP. The adverse reactions of hepatitis and neutropenia occurred less frequently than with TMP/SMX, while rash and GI upset occurred at the same rate. Mild hyperkalemia may be observed with trimethoprim / dapsone therapy (6).

Side Effects of Dapsone:

<u>Methemoglobinemia</u>. Almost all patients on dapsone will develop methemo-globin levels of 3-5%, without symptoms. For levels of greater than 10-15%, discontinue dapsone. For methemoglobin levels of 15-20%, especially in patients with respiratory compromise, consider treating with methylene blue.

<u>Hemolytic anemia</u> in patients with glucose-6-phosphate dehydrogenase deficiency.

"<u>Dapsone Syndrome</u>" consisting of rash, fever, and evidence of hepatic injury (jaundice, RUQ pain, hepatomegaly, or hyperbilirubinemia) has been reported in AIDS patients. Onset usually occurs after 3 - 8 weeks of therapy.

Management of Dapsone Therapy (with TMP or alone as prophylaxis):

-Check glucose-6-phosphate dehydrogenase (G6PD) level in all dark-skinned or Mediterranean patients before starting treatment. G6PD deficiency is present in 10-15% of African- American males, and a particularly severe variant is also found in patients of eastern Mediterranean (including Jewish) ancestry. As this trait is X-linked recessive, hemolysis is much less frequent in females. G6PD deficiency is rare in patients of Northern European descent.

-Suspect methemoglobinemia in any patient whose oxygen saturation by oximetry is lower than calculated from the PaO2 on ABG's, or whose pulse oximeter reading tends towards 85% without clinical explanation. 100% methemoglobin will read artifactually as 85% SaO2 on most pulse oximeters. The observed reading in methemoglobinemia will be a weighted average of this value and the percentage of normal oxyhemoglobin (13).

-The patient should not take the anti-viral agent dideoxyinosine (DDI) within 2 hours of dapsone, as the alkaline buffer in DDI will interfere with the absorption of dapsone.

4) Investigational drug:

BW566C80 (atovaquone), a hydroxynapthaquinone with anti-pneumocystis activity, is available on a compassionate-use basis from Burroughs Wellcome (1-800-755-2020) or local investigators for patients failing established therapy for PCP. The recommended dose is 750 mg po tid, immediately after meals, for 21 days (ref. 16).

c) Adjunctive Corticosteroids

Drug-induced damage to the pneumocystis organism is thought to exacerbate the pulmonary inflammatory response, adversely affecting alveolar function. Based on the findings of several studies (12), the San Francisco General Hospital (SFGH) PCP study group made the following recommendations (July, 1990) for corticosteroid use in PCP:

A. Patients with suspected PCP and room air pO2 > 70 mm Hg do not require corticosteroids.

B. Patients with severe PCP and room air pO2 < 50 mm Hg will likely benefit from adjuvant corticosteroids.

C. Patients presenting with moderately severe PCP and pO2 > 50 but < 70 must be individually assessed. Risks (coinfection, pneumothorax, ulcer disease) must be weighed against possible benefits of corticosteroid use. In addition, the clinical presentation of the patient, laboratory markers for disease severity, and the tempo of the disease process should be weighed before deciding to add steroids.

D. If adjunctive corticosteroid therapy is elected, steroids should be instituted coincident with institution of anti-PCP therapy.

In practice, it appears that steroids may be beneficial if begun within 72 hours of anti-PCP therapy, but have not been shown to be of any benefit if started later, and, in fact, may predispose the patient to secondary opportunistic infections (17). Definitive diagnosis of PCP should follow institution of therapy within 72 hours, and steroids should be discontinued if pneumocystis is not histologically documented.

Corticosteroid therapy, as oral prednisone or IV methylprednisolone should be dosed as follows:

Day 1-5: 40 mg po or IV bid
Day 6-10: 40 mg po or IV qd
Day 11-21: Initially 20 mg po or IV qd, followed by tapering over 21 days
and discontinuation simultaneous with anti-PCP therapy.

d. Ventilatory Support (Adapted from J.D. Stansell, MD, ref.7):

Categories of Patients more likely to benefit from Ventilatory Therapy:

1. Patients in whom a histologic diagnosis of PCP has not been made or who have not received an adequate length (7-10 days) of appropriate anti-PCP therapy.
2. Patients with documented PCP and a treatable respiratory co-infection should be supported.
3. Patients whose condition deteriorates rapidly as a result of a diagnostic procedure can demonstrate rapidly reversible respiratory failure.

The decision to counsel against intubation can be difficult. Patients with histologically documented PCP, who develop respiratory failure despite 7-10 days of appropriate therapy, and without identifiable co-infection are unlikely to benefit from intubation and ventilatory support. Similarly, AIDS patients with a history of multiple opportunistic infections, neoplasms, or wasting syndrome frequently will not respond to antibiotic therapy. Each case must be evaluated with attention to the desires and best interests of the individual patient.

5. Outcome and Sequelae

With appropriate therapy, radiographic improvement and resolution of fever are expected after 7 to 10 days.

Pneumothorax occurs in 2-9% of patients with PCP. In addition to the infection itself, catheter placement, transbronchial biopsy, and PEEP may contribute to increased risk. Placement of a chest tube to vacuum, until no air leak is detected, is usually required. After the air leak has stopped, if the lung remains inflated after 4 hours on water seal, pleurodesis should be attempted. Occasionally, surgical repair is indicated following adequate therapy for PCP. Steroids should be discontinued in patients who develop a pneumothorax.

Survival of patients with mild to moderate episodes of PCP (PaO2 >70 mmHg or A-a gradient of <35 mm Hg) is generally >80%. More severe episodes have a poorer, but not hopeless, prognosis.

6. Prophylactic Therapy & Follow-up (18):

The spontaneous relapse rate of PCP following standard therapy is 35% at 6 months, and 60% at one year. Therefore, secondary prophylaxis against PCP is indicated in all patients following treatment. Primary prophylaxis is also indicated for HIV-positive patients with CD4 counts ≤200, as the chance of developing PCP is about 20% within one year after the CD4 count declines to

200. In patients with candidiasis or chronic fevers, prophylaxis may be initiated at somewhat higher CD4 counts.

-**The drug of choice for PCP prophylaxis** is trimethoprim/sulfamethoxazole (TMP/SMX), one double-strength tablet po daily or 3 days per week (optimal dosing has not been established). The failure rate in secondary prophylaxis is about 5% per year. A desensitization protocol has been proposed for patients with mild reactions to TMP/SMX; safety and efficacy are unknown (20).

-In patients who cannot tolerate TMP/SMX (rash, nausea, or leukopenia), aerosolized pentamidine, 300 mg via Respirgard II nebulizer q month, or 60 mg via Fisoneb nebulizer, 5 times in first 2 weeks and 60 mg q 2 wks thereafter, may be used. While systemic toxicity is low, the failure rate in secondary prophylaxis is about 20% per year, and there is no protection against systemic infection with PCP. There is increasing evidence that systemic therapies are generally superior.

-Dapsone, 50-100 mg po q day, shows promise as primary prophylaxis (19) and is currently in trials as secondary prophylaxis against PCP. G6PD levels should be checked before starting therapy (see section 4.b.2 under "Treatment" above). Pyrimethamine, 50 mg po q week, may be combined with dapsone (21).

Less frequently used regimens:

-Pyrimethamine sulfadoxine (Fansidar), 1 tablet q week, appears to provide effective prophylaxis against PCP, but is associated with significant risk of serious Stevens-Johnson syndrome; fatalities have occurred.

-Patients receiving pyrimethamine/sulfadiazine for chronic suppression of toxoplasmosis do not require additional prophylaxis against PCP (3).

-One study suggests that pyrimethamine/dapsone may provide effective primary prophylaxis against both PCP and toxoplasmosis (See ref. 12 of the chapter on toxoplasmosis).

-Parenteral pentamidine given monthly may prove to be a viable option. (S. Safrin, SFGH Medicine Grand Rounds, September 1992).

References

1) Goodman PC. The chest film in AIDS. In The Medical Management of AIDS, 2nd ed. Sande, MA and PA Volberding, eds. Saunders, 1990.

2) Farizo KM, et al. Spectrum of disease in persons with human immunodeficiency virus infection in the United States. JAMA 1992; 267:1798-1805.

3) Heald A, et al. Treatment for cerebral toxoplasmosis protects against Pneumocystis carinii pneumonia in patients with AIDS. Annals Int. Med. 1991; 115: 760-763.

4) Sepkowitz KA, et al. Pneumothorax in AIDS. Annals Int. Med 1991; 114 455-459.

5) McClellan MD, et al. Pneumothorax with Pneumocystis carinii pneumonia

AIDS. Chest 1991; 100:1224-1227.

6) Medina I, et al. Oral therapy for Pneumocystis carinii pneumonia in the acquired immune deficiency syndrome: a controlled trial of trimethoprim-sulfamethoxazole versus trimethoprim-dapsone. NEJM 1990; 323:776-782.

7) Stansell JD "Pneumocystis carinii pneumonia: history and diagnosis" and "Ventilatory support -- who will benefit?" in AIDSFILE 1991;5:1-3. Copyright 1991, The Regents of the University of California.

8) Zaman MK and DL White. Serum lactate dehydrogenase levels and Pneumocystis carinii pneumonia: diagnostic and prognostic significance. Annual Rev. Resp. Disease 1988; 137:796-800.

9) Naidich DP and G McGuinness. Pulmonary manifestations of AIDS. Radiology Clinics of N. America 1991; 29(S):997-1017.

10) Curtis J, et al. Noninvasive tests in the diagnostic evaluation for Pneumocystis carinii pneumonia in patients with or suspected of having AIDS. Annual Rev. Resp. Disease 1986; 133:A182.

11) Chaisson RE. Infections due to encapsulated bacteria, salmonella, shigella, and campylobacter. in The Medical Management of AIDS, 2nd ed. Volberding, PA and MA Sande, eds. Saunders, 1990.

12) The NIH-UC expert panel for corticosteroids as adjunctive therapy for Pneumocystis carinii pneumonia. Consensus statement on the use of corticosteroids as adjunctive therapy for Pneumocystis carinii pneumonia in the acquires immune deficiency syndrome. NEJM 1990; 323:1500-1504.

13) Ralston AC, et al. Potential errors in pulse oximetry III: Effects of interference, dyes, dyshaemoglobins and other pigments. Anaesthesia 1991; 46:291-295.

14) White DA and MK Zaman. Medical management of AIDS patients: Pulmonary disease. Medical Clinics of North America 1992; 45:163-168.

15) "Thoracic Manifestations of AIDS" Journal of Thoracic Imaging 1991, vol.6. Contributions by Goodman, Stansell, Daley, Conces and Tarver on pp 16-64.

16) Hughes WT. A new drug for the treatment of Pneumocystis carinii pneumonia. Annals of Internal Medicine 1992; 116:953-954.

17) Nelson M. Steroid treatment - an association with overt CMV disease in patients with AIDS. Abstr. PoB 3228, VIII Intl. Conf. on AIDS, Amsterdam 1992.

18) Centers For Disease Control. Recommendations for prophylaxis against Pneumocystis carinii pneumonia in adolescents and adults. JAMA 1992; 267:2294-2299.

19) Blum RW, et al. Comparative trial of dapsone versus TMP/SMX for primary prophylaxis of PCP. Journal of AIDS 1992; 5:341-347.

20) White, MV, et al. Desensitization to trimethoprim sulfamethoxazole in patients with the acquired immune deficiency syndrome and pneumocystis carinii pneumonia. Annals of Allergy 1989; 62:177-179.

21) Opravil M, et al. Combined prophylaxis of Pneumocystis carinii pneumonia and toxoplasmosis: prospective, randomized trial of dapsone + pyrimethamine vs. aerosolized pentamidine. Abstr. B139, VII Intl. Conf. on AIDS, Amsterdam 1992.

Toxoplasma gondii

1. Introduction

The protozoan Toxoplasma gondii is the most common cause of CNS mass lesions in patients with AIDS. Toxoplasma may also cause pneumonia, chorioretinitis, myocarditis, orchitis, peritonitis, and infection of the spinal cord (conus medullaris syndrome).

Toxoplasmosis occurs in about 4% of AIDS patients at the University of California, San Francisco (UCSF). Significantly higher risk has been reported in patients from the Caribbean basin, especially Haitians. Toxoplasma encephalitis occurs much more frequently among AIDS patients in France and Germany. The illness is thought to result from reactivation of previous infection.

The most common source of primary infection in humans is probably ingestion of raw or undercooked beef, lamb, or pork. Cats, which are the definitive host of Toxoplasma gondii, may transiently shed infectious oocysts in their feces (see section 6b below).

2. Presentation (2,5)

a) Toxoplasma encephalitis

History: Between 45% and 75% report headache, of mean duration 2 wks. Fever occurs in 35%. 50-70% of patients with cerebral toxoplasmosis present with disordered consciousness or cognition, ranging from mild dementia to coma. The average duration of mental status changes is 3 wks. The incidence of focal findings is also 70%, including hemi- or monoparesis (30%), seizures (25%) and ataxia (21%). Incontinence, hemi-sensory disturbances, isolated cranial nerve palsies, aphasia, and visual complaints each occur in approximately 10% of patients.

The CD4 count is usually <200 T-helper cells per microliter, and is frequently <50.

Physical Exam: Frank meningeal signs are rare, and if present, another cause should be considered. Especially common findings include focal neurological findings such as hemiparesis, visual field defects, and cerebellar findings.

Imaging: MRI, if available, is the imaging method of choice. CT scanning reveals multiple mass lesions, usually bilateral, in 70% of affected patients. 20% have a single lesion, and 10% show no focal finding on CT. MRI is more sensitive than CT, revealing lesions not seen on CT scan in approximately 25% of cases. MRI is especially important if only one lesion is seen on CT, because detection of additional lesions on MRI argues strongly for toxoplasmosis, while a lesion confirmed by MRI to be solitary is more likely to represent a primary

CNS lymphoma, tuberculoma, or fungal abscess.

Lesions are usually contrast-enhancing, but may be low-density or nodular in appearance. Edema surrounding each lesion is common. Toxoplasmosis abscesses tend to respect anatomical boundaries, so that lesions crossing gyral borders are more likely to be due to lymphoma. Anatomical locations of cerebral toxoplasmosis lesions include basal ganglia (most frequent), parietal, frontal, and occipital lobes, and posterior fossa (least frequent).

Differential diagnosis of focal CNS lesions:

The following table shows the comparative incidence of CNS mass lesions in AIDS patients. As this data was assembled in the mid-1980's, infections associated with intravenous drug use, such as bacterial abscesses and tuberculosis, are probably under-represented.

Stroke should also be considered in evaluating focal neurologic deficits in HIV-positive patients, as the incidence of cerebrovascular occlusive disease (usually idiopathic) is approximately 300 times higher in this population than in age-matched controls (5).

Histopathologic diagnosis in AIDS patients with focal CNS lesions on CT (1)

Diagnosis	% of Patients in series	% of all UCSF AIDS patients with this diagnosis
Toxoplasmosis	50-70%	4%
Primary CNS Lymphoma	10-25%	2%
Progressive multi-focal leukoencephalopathy	10-22%	0.6%
Candida abscess	3%	
Cryptococcoma	2%	
Kaposi's sarcoma	2%	
M. tuberculosis abscess	1%	
Herpes simplex II	1%	
Non-diagnostic	10%	

Labs:

Serum toxoplasmosis titer is non-specific and of limited sensitivity, as only about 25-35% of AIDS patients with toxoplasmosis antibodies actually develop toxoplasmosis, and 15-20% of patients with biopsy-proven toxoplasmosis at San Francisco General Hospital (SFGH) have negative toxoplasmosis titers. There is evidence, however, that an **increase** in serum anti-toxoplasma IgG titer is associated with the development of cerebral toxoplasmosis (6).

Cerebrospinal fluid analysis, if performed, is non-specific. Protein may be moderately increased to around 100 mg/dl. Glucose may be normal or slightly decreased. Cells average 6 lymphocytes per microliter and rarely exceed 70. CSF is normal in 20% of cases.

CNS toxoplasmosis titer is not usually performed. This test adds little diagnostic information, as IgG crosses the blood-brain barrier from serum, and IgM is not usually present in reactivated infection.

b) Ocular toxoplasmosis must be distinguished from CMV retinitis, especially in populations with high rates of toxoplasma infection. Active lesions consist of homogeneous, yellow-white, edematous regions of necrotizing retinitis, usually accompanied by overlying vitreal inflammation, with frequent inflammation of the anterior segment as well. If untreated, lesions progress to destroy the entire retina. In one study, 29% of patients with ocular toxoplasmosis had a concurrent cerebral focus, 9% had a prior diagnosis of toxoplasma encephalitis, and 9% later developed brain involvement (8).

c) Toxoplasma pneumonia is rare, accounting for <1% of AIDS pneumonias (4). Affected patients usually have CD4 count <100 T-helper cells/microliter. Presentation includes fever, dyspnea, hypoxia and bilateral pulmonary infiltrates or nodular densities. Diagnosis consists of detecting tachyzoites on broncho--alveolar lavage.

3. Treatment of Toxoplasmosis Infections:

Given the uncertainty of laboratory diagnosis, most clinicians will treat suspected toxoplasmosis empirically. Hollander (5) recommends that definitive diagnosis by stereotactic brain biopsy should be offered without the delay of empirical treatment in the following settings: 1) a solitary lesion on MRI, 2) intolerance to therapeutic agents for toxoplasmosis, 3) rapid neurologic deterioration, and 4) cerebral edema that necessitates the use of corticosteroids, which may partially treat CNS lymphoma, thereby confusing the results of brain biopsy and obscuring the effects of therapy on follow-up imaging studies.

a) Treatment of choice (pyrimethamine + sulfadiazine):

Pyrimethamine, 50-100 mg po qd following a loading dose of 200 mg po on day 1, plus sulfadiazine, 4-6 grams po per day in 4 divided doses. Duration of acute treatment is usually 4-8 weeks, depending on clinical response.

Side Effects of Pyrimethamine:

Rash, sometimes progressing to Stevens-Johnson syndrome.

Rash is a common side effect of all current treatment regimens for toxoplasmosis. If neutropenia, elevated liver transaminases, or Stevens-Johnson syndrome accompany rash, therapy should be changed. If none of these conditions is present, consider treating rash with antihistamines or antipruritics, or both, with careful monitoring of patient.

Myelosuppression, including leukopenia, thrombocytopenia, or megaloblastic anemia.
GI disturbances, including vomiting, diarrhea, abdominal cramps.

Management of Pyrimethamine Therapy:

-Folinic acid (Leucovorin), 10 mg po qd, should be given to counteract the myelosuppressive effect of pyrimethamine. The dose may be increased to as much as 50 mg qd in response to developing neutropenia.
-Folate supplements should not be given, as they will interfere with the therapeutic action of pyrimethamine.

Side effects of sulfadiazine:

Rash, sometimes progressing to Stevens-Johnson syndrome.
Myelosuppression, including leukopenia, thrombocytopenia, and megaloblastic anemia.
Crystalluria, sometimes leading to nephropathy and acute renal failure.
GI disturbances, including nausea, vomiting, and abdominal pain.

Management of Sulfadiazine Therapy:

-Avoid urine acidifying agents, such as high-dose vitamin C, as they increase the risk of crystalluria.
-Keep the patient well hydrated at all times to prevent crystalluria.

b) Alternative Toxoplasmosis Treatments:

1) In patients with sulfonamide sensitivity, pyrimethamine (at the above doses) may be combined with clindamycin, 450-600 mg po qid, or 600-900 mg IV q 6 hrs. Side effects of clindamycin are less frequent than those of sulfadiazine, and include rash, nausea, vomiting, diarrhea, and pseudomembranous colitis.

2) BW566C80 (atovaquone), an experimental hydroxynaphthaquinone with activity against pneumocystis and toxoplasma (7), is available from the manufacturer (Burroughs Wellcome (1-800-755-2020) or local investigators on a compassionate-use basis for patients failing standard therapy. This drug has been used in salvage therapy, and may act synergistically with other anti-toxoplasma agents (13,14). 566C80 is often given in combination with pyrimethamine.

c) <u>**Corticosteroids**</u> (eg, dexamethasone (Decadron), 4 mg q 6 hrs) are used as adjunctive therapy in patients with cerebral edema on MRI or CT and any of the following:
1) Altered mental status
2) Midline shift or danger of herniation
3) Active seizures on presentation.

d) <u>**Mannitol**</u>, 1.5-2 gm/kg IV, can be given if signs of herniation are present.

4. Outcome and Sequelae of Toxoplasmosis Therapy: (5)

Most patients begin to show clinical improvement within one week of starting therapy. In these patients CT or MRI should be repeated 2-3 weeks after the initiation of therapy. Radiographic improvement is seen in 70% of patients with toxoplasmosis after 2 weeks, and in approximately 90% after 3 weeks of treatment. The earliest finding is a decrease in edema around the lesions; thus the use of corticosteroids may confuse the results of empiric anti-toxoplasmosis therapy. If lesions are worse or unchanged following 2-3 weeks of therapy, biopsy should be offered.

If clinical deterioration occurs, imaging studies should be repeated before 2-3 weeks of treatment. If worsening of edema or an increase in the size or number of lesions is detected, then biopsy should be considered, if in the best interest of the patient.

Following successful treatment of toxoplasmosis, some patients will have a lowered seizure threshold, possibly due to glial scarring, and these patients may require continued anticonvulsant therapy.

5. Maintenance Therapy

While the initial response rate of toxoplasmosis to antimicrobial therapy is about 85%, some 30-50% of patients will relapse once therapy is discontinued. For this reason, lifelong maintenance therapy is required once clinical and radiographic resolution have occurred.

-Chronic suppression is achieved with pyrimethamine, 25 mg po qd or 50 mg po qod, plus either:
Clindamycin, 300 mg po qid, or
Sulfadiazine, 500 mg - 1 g po qid.
-Folinic acid, 5-10 mg po qd should be included in chronic therapy to prevent myelotoxicity.

6. Prevention of Toxoplasmosis

a) Prophylactic therapy

The status of primary prophylaxis against toxoplasmosis has not been established. Given the frequency with which toxoplasma-infected patients develop disease, however, many physicians will prophylactically treat HIV-infected patients with positive toxoplasma titers and CD4 count <200. There is evidence that trimethoprim-sulfamethoxazole given as secondary PCP prophylaxis is protective against toxoplasmosis (10, 11). Pyrimethamine-dapsone (12), azithromycin, and 566C80 (atovaquone) have shown promise in early studies, and pyrimethamine-sulfadiazine- leucovorin given two days per week at maintenance doses is sometimes used.

A recent NIH-sponsored, community-based study of primary prophylaxis with pyrimethamine alone in patients with CD4 count <200 and a positive toxoplasmosis titer was discontinued due to increased mortality in the group receiving prophylaxis (M Jacobson, personal communication, 1992). Clindamycin alone produces a high rate of dose-limiting diarrhea (9).

b) Toxoplasma in Pet Cats:

The likelihood of infection in a pet cat is diminished by keeping the animal indoors, feeding it commercial cat food, and not allowing it to eat birds, rodents, or raw meat. Oocysts shed in feces are not infectious until at least 24 hours after defecation. Litter boxes should therefore be changed daily, preferably by a non-HIV-infected individual. HIV-infected individuals should wear a mask and gloves if they must change cat boxes.

References

1) De La Paz RL and D Enzmann. Neuroradiology of AIDS. In Rosenblum et al, eds., <u>AIDS and the Nervous System</u>. New York, Raven Press, 1988.

2) Levy RM and DE Bredesen. Central nervous system dysfunction in AIDS. In Rosenblum et al, eds., <u>AIDS and the Nervous System</u>. New York, Raven Press, 1988.

3) Danneman B, et al. Treatment of toxoplasmic encephalitis in patients with AIDS. Annals of Internal Medicine 1992; 116:33-43.

4) Oksenhendler E, et al. Toxoplasma gondii pneumonia in patients with the acquired immune deficiency syndrome. American Journal of Medicine 1990; 88:18N-25N.

5) Hollander H. Neurologic and psychiatric manifestations of HIV disease. Journal of General Internal Medicine 1991; 6(suppl.):S24-S31.

6) Sugar A. Serology of latent toxoplasmic infection and cerebral toxoplasmosis in patients from the Swiss HIV cohort study. Abstr. PoB 3264, VIII Intl. Conf. on AIDS, Amsterdam 1992.

7) Araujo FG. In vitro and in vivo activities of the hydroxynaphthoquinone 566C80 against the cyst form of Toxoplasma gondii. Antimicrobial Agents and Chemotherapy 1992; 36:326.

8) Cochereau-Massin I, et al. Ocular toxoplasmosis in HIV-infected patients. American Journal of Ophthalmology 1992; 114:130-135.

9) Jacobson MA. Toxicity of clindamycin as prophylaxis for AIDS-associated toxoplasmic encephalitis. Lancet 1992; 339:333.

10) Carr A, et al. Low-dose trimethoprim-sulfamethoxazole prophylaxis for PCP found to protect against toxoplasmic encephalitis in patients with AIDS. Annals

of Internal Medicine 1992; 117:106-111.
11) Schneider M. Efficacy of aerosolized pentamidine and low dose co-trimoxazole for primary prevention of PCP. Abstr. WeB 1018, VIII Intl. Conf. on AIDS, Amsterdam 1992.
12) Girard PM, et al. Dapsone-pyrimethamine versus aerosolized pentamidine for primary prophylaxis of pneumocystis and neurotoxoplasmosis. Abstr. WeB 1017, VIII Intl. Conf. on AIDS, Amsterdam 1992.
13) Grundman M. Neuroradiologic response to 566C80 salvage therapy for CNS toxoplasmosis. Abstr. PoB 3185; VIII Intl. Conf. on AIDS, Amsterdam, 1992.
14) Kovacs JA. Evaluation of azithromycin or the combination of 566C80 and pyrimethamine in the treatment of cerebral toxoplasmosis. Abstr. PoB 3199. VII Intl. Conf. on AIDS, Amsterdam 1992.

Cryptococcus neoformans

1. Introduction

Infection with the fungus Cryptococcus neoformans causes serious illness in approximately 8% of AIDS patients in the United States. Cryptococcal meningitis accounts for some 80% of these cases, with disseminated cryptococcemia and pulmonary cryptococcosis occurring less frequently. Disseminated infection may involve the skin, presenting as umbilicated papules resembling molluscum. The prostate may harbor chronic infection in treated patients.

The fungus is found worldwide.   Pigeon droppings and soil are common reservoirs of infection.

2. Presentation of Cryptococcal Infection

a. Cryptococcal Meningitis (2,3)

History: Frequently cryptococcal meningitis is the first opportunistic infection to occur in HIV-infected patients. Onset may be subtle, with preclinical course including fever and night sweats. 85% of patients report headache which is often mild and of average duration of 11 days.   About one-third report impaired consciousness or cognition, often of 2-3 wks duration. Photophobia occurs in <25%, seizures in <15%.

CD_4 count is usually <100 T-helper cells per microliter.

The differential diagnosis of headache in HIV-positive patients must include migraine and tension headache, as well as sinusitis, an especially common problem in this patient population. Headache is also reported by 43-73% of patients with cerebral toxoplasmosis.

Physical Exam: Often unrevealing. Frank meningismus is present in only one-third of patients. Focal neurologic findings are unusual.

Imaging: In patients with altered mental status, obtundation, seizures, or focal neurologic findings, CT or MRI should be performed, before lumbar puncture is performed, to rule out mass lesions (often due to toxoplasmosis or CNS lymphoma). CT is usually negative or nonspecific in cryptococcal meningitis, but cryptococcoma may be seen in 12% of patients. Meningeal enhancement is unusual, occurring in <10%. Communicating or non-communicating hydrocephalus is occasionally found, and should be treated (section 3c, below).

Labs:
Serum cryptococcal antigen (CrAg) is 99% sensitive. In the absence of prior treatment for cryptococcal infection, a titer as low as 1:2 should be considered

positive and representative of a site of active infection. 87% of patients with cryptococcal meningitis will have a serum CrAg of 1:32 or higher. False negatives have been reported in 1%. Rare false positive may occur in the presence of rheumatoid factor or infection with Trichosporum beigeii.
 -In the patient who has received prior treatment for cryptococcus, relapse should be suspected if CrAg titers have increased by greater than 2 to 4 fold.

<u>CSF indices</u> are nonspecific and may be near normal in cryptococcal meningitis:

-Opening pressure is usually elevated, exceeding 200 mm H20 in two-thirds of patients. Patients with markedly elevated opening pressure should undergo CT or MRI to rule out communicating hydrocephalus.
-Glucose is depressed in only one-fourth of patients (average 43 mg/dl).
-Protein is elevated in about one-half of patients, but rarely exceeds 150 mg/dl (average 82 mg/dl).
-Cell count typically shows mild lymphocytic pleocytosis. Only 20% of patients have >20 WBC/microliter, and WBC counts exceeding 200/microliter are rare.

<u>India ink staining</u> is 80% sensitive for detecting cryptococcus in CSF. Specificity is near 100%. However, the presence of cryptococcus in the CSF may persist during the first 2 months of treatment and does not indicate treatment failure during this period (JD Stansell, personal communication, 1992).
<u>CSF CrAg</u> is 91% sensitive, apparently less sensitive than serum CrAg. Titers are 1:32 or higher in 71% of patients with confirmed cryptococcal meningitis.
<u>Blood and CSF Cryptococcus cultures</u> should be sent to confirm diagnosis.

Differential Diagnosis of Cerebrospinal Fluid Abnormalities:

HIV infection alone may cause increased CSF protein of up to 80 mg/dl, with as many as 10-30 monocytes, and normal glucose, in as many as one-third of asymptomatic individuals with early HIV disease. Headaches and even cranial nerve palsies may be associated with this syndrome. As disease advances and CD4 counts fall, pleocytosis is less common, but moderate elevation in CSF protein persists. For CSF protein >100 or WBC>30, however, some other cause must be sought.

In addition to infection with cryptococcus or HIV alone, the differential diagnosis of lymphocytic pleocytosis in HIV disease includes tuberculous meningitis, neurosyphilis, fungal meningitides (coccidioides, histoplasma), viral CNS infection (herpes simplex types 1 and 2, varicella zoster), chronic inflammatory demyelinating polyneuropathy, lymphomatous meningitis, and parameningeal processes, especially intracranial mass lesions. (9).

Tuberculous meningitis deserves special emphasis, as Mycobacterium tuberculosis is isolated from CSF in 10% of HIV patients with pulmonary TB (versus 2% in HIV-negative controls). TB is thus a more frequent cause of meningitis than cryptococcus in HIV patients from populations in which TB is endemic. A recent study (10) found clinical manifestations of TB meningitis in HIV infection to be similar to those seen in HIV-negative patients. Common findings included fever >38 degrees (present in 81% of affected patients), headache (60%), meningeal signs (65%) and altered mental status (43%). About half of affected patients had pulmonary infiltrates suggestive of TB. CSF showed decreased glucose (85%), increased protein (57%), and lymphocytic pleocytosis (avg. 234 cells per cu mm [higher than usually observed in cryptococcal meningitis]; 90% had >5 lymphs). 22% had positive AFB smear of CSF. CT was abnormal in 70%, due to hydrocephalus (42%), focal lesions (43%), or meningeal enhancement (23%).

If a neutrophilic pleocytosis is present, bacterial meningitis or cytomegalovirus infection of the CNS (see chapter on CMV) should be considered. Reports of bacterial meningitis due to common pathogens are few in AIDS patients, suggesting that AIDS patients are not at appreciably higher risk for these infections. Moreover, Listeria monocytogenes, the most common cause of bacterial meningitis in patients immunosuppressed for reasons other than HIV infection, is a rare cause of meningitis in AIDS. Additionally, nocardia meningitis, which frequently complicates pulmonary infection with Nocardia asteroides in other immunocompromised patients, is extremely rare in AIDS (5).

b. Cryptococcal Pneumonia:

Pulmonary infection with cryptococcus tends to cause diffuse infiltrates on chest X-ray mimicking PCP. Pleural effusion, which is rare in PCP, may be present. Intrathoracic lymphadenopathy, nodular infiltrates that may cavitate, and even normal chest X-ray have also been reported. CD4 count is usually <200.

Since 13% of patients presenting with cryptococcal meningitis will also have PCP, diagnosis of pulmonary disease should proceed as described in that chapter.

3. Treatment of Cryptococcal Meningitis (1,6,7):

Anti-cryptococcal therapy should be started for patients with a clinical presentation, elevated serum CrAg, and CSF findings indicative of cryptococcal meningitis without awaiting culture results.

Cryptococcal meningitis findings indicating high risk for early deterioration and death (6):
1) Altered mental status (lethargy, somnolence or obtundation) on presen-

tation;
2) CSF CrAg titer higher than 1:1024
3) Patients with normal mental status, CSF CrAg higher than 1:1024, and CSF WBC>20 appeared to be at low risk, despite elevated CSF CrAg. Serum CrAg was not found to predict outcome.

a) <u>Low-risk Patients</u>

Meningitis patients at low risk (normal mental status <u>and</u> CSF CrAg titer 1:1024 or lower), may be treated from the outset with fluconazole, 400 mg po qd for 10-12 weeks, and followed closely. Outpatient treatment is possible if the patient is reliable, able to keep appointments, and has a person to monitor the patient at home.

Fluconazole is generally well tolerated. Side effects include nausea, vomiting, abdominal pain, diarrhea, headache, and elevated transaminases. Concurrent treatment with rifampin tends to decrease levels of fluconazole. Fluconazole may increase the activity of phenytoin, warfarin, and the sulfonylureas.

b) <u>High-risk patients</u>

Optimal treatment for patients at high risk (due to <u>either</u> altered mental status or CSF CrAg higher than 1:1024) has not been determined.

1) Most clinicians at San Francisco General Hospital feel that a reasonable approach is to start with amphotericin B, 0.5-0.8 mg/kg IV q day, infused over 2-4 hrs.

2) Patients with adequate WBC may be treated with amphotericin B, 0.5-0.8 mg/kg/d IV, plus flucytosine, 25 mg/kg po q 6 hrs.

Treatment with amphotericin, with or without flucytosine, should continue until definite symptomatic and clinical improvement is noted, usually at least 1 to 2 weeks. Thereafter, treatment may be switched to fluconazole, 400 mg po qd, to complete a full 10-12 week course of therapy. Alternatively, amphotericin may be continued to a total dose of 2.5 grams.

<u>Side effects of Amphotericin B:</u>

<u>Fever and chills:</u> common. May be improved by premedicating with aspirin (600 mg po) or acetaminophen 30 minutes prior to infusion. Hydrocortisone, 25 mg mixed with each dose, may also reduce side effects. If these are ineffective, meperidine (Demerol), 50 mg IV, may be used to premedicate. Meperidine, 25 mg IV, may also be used to shorten the duration of a rigor already in progress. Fevers, which may exceed 40 degrees C, tend to

diminish after the first several infusions.

Nausea and vomiting: May be improved by premedicating with an antiemetic.

Hypokalemia: Supplement if K falls to 3.8 or below.

Hypomagnesemia: Supplement as needed.

Nephrotoxicity: Serum creatinine will rise in >80% of patients. RTA and nephrocalcinosis are also observed. If creatinine rises above 2.5 mg/dl, reduce dose or discontinue amphotericin until creatinine returns to 1.5 or less.

Anemia: Normocytic and normochromic, probably due to impairment of erythropoietin function. Reversible with termination of treatment.

Thrombophlebitis: occurs at infusion site. May add heparin, 500 to 1,000 U to each infusion as prophylaxis.

Management of Amphotericin B Therapy:

-The traditional 1 mg "test dose" is not necessary, as anaphylaxis is rare (8). Typically, treatment is begun as a 10-20 mg infusion given over 4 hours. The patient is observed, with monitoring of vital signs over the first 15-20 minutes. If no serious reaction is observed, the infusion is continued.
-In critically ill AIDS patients requiring amphotericin, there is no benefit expected from gradually increasing the dose over several days. In these patients, a 20 mg infusion is started with monitoring as above. If this is tolerated, the balance of the desired daily dose may be given later the same day. In the absence of serious reaction, the full dose may then be given on day 2 and thereafter.
-Nephrotoxic effect is potentiated by volume depletion, often resulting from poor oral intake or vomiting. Giving normal saline, 500 cc IV over 30 min, before and after each infusion is recommended as a protective measure.
-Monitor CBC, creatinine, electrolytes (especially K, bicarbonate) and Mg at least qod.

Side Effects of Flucytosine:

The major toxicity of flucytosine is myelosuppression, leading to leukopenia, thrombocytopenia, or both. As this side effect is frequently dose-limiting in AIDS patients, flucytosine at SFGH is reserved for use in patients with severe disease and adequate WBC. Other side effects include nausea, vomiting, diarrhea, elevated liver enzymes, and rash.

If a decision is made to treat with flucytosine, CBC with differential and platelets should be monitored daily. Serum creatinine should also be monitored closely, as flucytosine is renally excreted, and impairment of renal function occurring with amphotericin therapy will lead to increased myelotoxicity due to increased serum flucytosine levels.

c) <u>Hydrocephalus</u>:

Patients with communicating hydrocephalus on CT or MRI should receive acetazolamide, 250 mg qid. Severe cases may require additional treatment with dexamethasone (Decadron), 4 mg q 6 hrs (J.D. Stansell, personal communication). Non-communicating hydrocephalus may require shunt placement.

4. Extra-neural cryptococcosis:

Fluconazole, 400 mg po qd for 6-10 weeks, may be used in treating extra-neural cryptococcal infection, as indicated by positive serum CrAg or blood culture in the absence of meningitis or pulmonary involvement. Chronic suppression (see 6a below) should then be continued for life.

Patients with severe cryptococcal pulmonary involvement should receive the same treatment as high-risk meningitis patients.

5. Outcome of Cryptococcal Meningitis Therapy:

Clinical improvement occurs over several weeks. Serum CrAg titers may rise by two- to four-fold during the first 4 to 6 weeks of therapy, and cannot be used to monitor treatment success in this setting (J.D. Stansell, personal communication). Confirmation of successful treatment rests on conversion of blood and CSF cryptococcus cultures to negative. These cultures are usually repeated after 10-12 weeks of therapy. If cultures are negative, the patient is changed to maintenance therapy (see below). If blood or CSF culture is positive, treatment with amphotericin or fluconazole is continued at full treatment doses, with repeat cultures 2-4 weeks later. Following treatment for cryptococcal meningitis, CSF and serum CrAg titers may remain elevated despite negative follow-up cultures, and are not thought to indicate active disease in this setting. An increasing serum CrAg following 6-8 weeks of treatment, however, suggests treatment failure or recurrence of active disease.

Mortality due to progressive cryptococcal disease in treated patients is 10-20%. In high-risk patients (see section 3 above), mortality is 30-40%.

6. Maintenance and Follow-up Therapy after Cryptococcal Infection:

a) Maintenance therapy after Cryptococcal Meningitis:

The recurrence rate of cryptococcal disease is 50-60%, and life expectancy is decreased, in patients not receiving suppressive therapy following initial treatment for cryptococcal meningitis. Lifelong maintenance therapy is therefore recommended once negative serum and CSF cryptococcus cultures have been documented at the completion of primary treatment.

-The treatment of choice for chronic suppression of treated cryptococcal meningitis is fluconazole, 200 mg po qd. 97% of patients receiving this therapy in a recent study remained relapse-free at one year, and side effects were few (4).

-The previous standard of care, amphotericin B, 1 mg/kg IV q week, showed a relapse-free rate of only 78% at one year, with a significantly higher rate of drug-related toxicity and bacterial infection, possibly related to the use of IV catheters.

b) Prophylaxis against Cryptococcal Infection:

The question of primary prophylaxis against cryptococcal meningitis has not been studied extensively. It has been suggested that fluconazole, 100 mg po qd (or 200 mg po qod) may be appropriate in any HIV patient with fewer than 100 T-helper cells/microliter, but there is inadequate evidence to recommend this approach at present, as the possibility exists that such treatment may select for drug-resistant strains.

Patients with CD4 counts < 100-200 should be monitored frequently for conversion of serum CrAg titers to positive, and treatment (sec. 4 above) should be started promptly if such conversion occurs.

References

1) Terrell CL and CE Hughes. Antifungal agents used for deep-seated mycotic infections. Mayo Clinic Proceedings 1992; 67:69-91.

2) Clement M. Cryptococcal disease: an update. AIDSFILE 1991; 5:1-2.

3) Chuck SL and MA Sande. Infections with Cryptococus neoformans in the acquired immune deficiency syndrome. NEJM 1989; 321:794-799.

4) Powderly WG, et al. A controlled trial of fluconazole or amphotericin B to prevent relapse of cryptococcal meningitis in patients with the acquired immune deficiency syndrome. NEJM 1992; 326:793-798.

5) Levy RM, et al. Neurologic complications of HIV infection. American family physician 1990; 41:517-536.

6) Saag MS, et al. Comparison of amphotericin B with fluconazole in the treatment of acute AIDS-associated cryptococcal meningitis. NEJM 1992; 326:83-89.

7) The Medical Letter on Drugs and Therapeutics. Drugs for AIDS and associated infections. The Medical Letter 1191; 33:95-101.

8) Savosi GI. Amphotericin B: Still the gold standard for antifungal therapy. Postgraduate medicine 1990; 88:151-166.

9) Hollander H. Neurologic and Psychiatric manifestations of HIV disease. Journal of General Internal Medicine 1991; 6(suppl.):S24-S31.

10) Berenguer J, et al. Tuberculous meningitis in patients infected with the human immunodeficiency virus. NEJM 1992; 326:668-672.

Cytomegalovirus

1. Introduction

Cytomegalovirus (CMV) is the most common life-threatening viral opportunistic agent in AIDS. CMV infection is present in the majority of AIDS patients, and end-organ disease occurs in 10-30%. Common manifestations include retinitis, esophagitis, and intestinal involvement. Less frequent diagnoses include encephalitis, hepatitis, cholangitis, pancreatitis, pneumonia, and peripheral neuropathy. Adrenalitis is a common finding on autopsy, and may account in part for the adrenal insufficiency commonly observed in AIDS patients.

At San Francisco General Hospital, CMV retinitis was diagnosed in 5.7% of AIDS patients, and CMV esophagitis in 2.2%, in 1986 (2). Other centers have reported higher incidences.

2. Presentation of Cytomegalovirus Infection:

CMV disease is rarely seen in patients with CD4 count >100 T-helper cells per microliter.

a) <u>CMV retinitis</u>:

History: Often asymptomatic until the disease is well established. Common complaints include visual field defects, floaters, blurred vision, or decreased visual acuity. Symptoms usually begin unilaterally, but may come to involve both eyes if untreated. Eye pain is absent.

Physical Exam: One or several retinal lesions. Initially, these are small white areas with granular, irregular borders, which enlarge if untreated into fluffy, white exudates, often with associated hemorrhages.

Labs: Blood and urine CMV cultures are neither specific nor very sensitive. CMV can be isolated from the majority of patients with advanced AIDS, and 10-20% of individuals with newly diagnosed CMV retinitis will have negative blood and urine culture for CMV. Cultures may be useful, however, in monitoring efficacy of antiviral therapy, and especially in detecting antiviral drug resistance (7).

Differential Diagnosis of Retinal Lesions (1):

<u>AIDS retinopathy</u> is a benign condition present in >50% of AIDS patients, characterized by "cotton-wool spots" -- small, fluffy, white retinal lesions, sometimes associated with small retinal hemorrhages. Cotton-wool spots have regular borders and are rarely larger than one disk diameter in size.

They may at times be difficult to distinguish from early CMV lesions. Diagnosis is made easier by the fact that cotton-wool spots will resolve over a few weeks, while untreated CMV lesions will expand.

<u>Toxoplasmosis chorioretinitis</u> (see chapter on toxoplasmosis) is characterized by homogeneous, yellow-white, edematous retinal lesions with fluffy borders. In general, retinal lesions caused by toxoplasma are accompanied by overlying vitreitis and inflammation of the anterior segment, neither of which is usual in CMV retinitis. Also, toxoplasmic lesions are not usually hemorrhagic, while retinal hemorrhages are common in CMV infection (21). This is a much less common entity than CMV retinitis, but should be considered in patients infected with toxoplasma.

<u>Disseminated PCP</u> may produce multiple yellow plaque-like zones in the posterior pole.

<u>Herpes simplex and varicella zoster</u> viruses occasionally infect the retina.

<u>Cryptococcal chorioretinitis</u> may appear as bilateral, multi-focal choroidal infiltrates with retinal hemorrhages in patients with cryptococcal meningitis.

<u>Roth spots</u> may be present in intravenous drug users.

<u>Ocular syphilis</u> is rarely seen in AIDS.

b) <u>Cytomegalovirus Esophagitis</u> (6)

History: Most patients experience pain on swallowing (odynophagia), with or without mechanical difficulty in swallowing (dysphagia). Patients find odynophagia more troubling than dysphagia, and dysphagia generally does not occur in patients not reporting odynophagia. Epigastric pain not associated with swallowing occurs in about one-half of affected patients. Weight loss occurs in one-third. Symptoms average one month in duration prior to presentation.

Physical Exam: Diagnosis is by endoscopy. Large (>10 cm^2), shallow ulcers are usually visualized in affected patients.

Labs: Biopsy specimens should be stained for intranuclear inclusion bodies (highly sensitive) and cultured to rule out candida and herpes simplex. CMV culture of biopsy specimens is only 50% sensitive.

Differential Diagnosis of Esophageal Lesions:

<u>Candida esophagitis</u> usually presents as dysphagia, rather than odynophagia. Patients commonly complain of food "sticking." Oral thrush is usually, but not always, present. Barium radiograph usually shows diffuse plaques and shallow ulcerations in the esophageal mucosa (9). Ketoconazole, 200-400 mg po qd, or fluconazole, 100-200 mg po qd, may be given empirically in these patients, with endoscopy only if this treatment fails.

<u>Herpes esophagitis</u> is similar to CMV in clinical presentation, causing retro-sternal pain, odynophagia and dysphagia. Endoscopy reveals multiple

ulcers that are deeper and smaller than CMV ulcers, surrounded by edematous, erythematous mucosa ("volcano ulcers") from which HSV is cultured. Treatment is with acyclovir, or foscarnet in acyclovir-resistant cases (10).

Aphthous ulcers of the esophagus also cause odynophagia and dysphagia in patients with HIV. Endoscopy reveals 2-15 mm ulcers that may resemble CMV ulcers but are negative for CMV on biopsy stain and culture. In some cases, HIV is isolated from these lesions, suggesting a possible etiologic role (10). Treatment with prednisone (40 mg qd for 1 week, followed by taper over the next 3 weeks) is sometimes effective (22). Thalidomide (100 mg bid) has also been reported to be effective against idiopathic oropharyngeal and esophageal ulcerations in AIDS (23).

The antiretroviral drug ddC (zalcitabine) may cause esophageal ulceration.

c) CMV Colitis: (2,11,14):

Colitis is thought to be the most common enteric disease caused by CMV in AIDS patients, occurring more frequently than CMV esophagitis, gastritis, or small intestinal enteritis.

History: Diarrhea, fever, and abdominal pain, intermittent and cramp-like, occasionally continuous. Hematochezia is not unusual. Most patients have a long, indolent course of symptoms, although rapidly progressive disease leading to colonic perforation or hemorrhagic colitis does occur.

Physical Exam: Colonoscopy (performed if laboratory workup is negative) may range from localized hyperemia to hemorrhagic erythema to superficial or deep ulceration.

Labs: Mucosal biopsy reveals intranuclear inclusion bodies and no other etiology for symptoms.

Blood and urine CMV cultures are of low sensitivity (30% and 70%, respectively), and low specificity.

Stool cultures for CMV are not helpful.

Differential Diagnosis of Diarrhea:

Diarrhea complicates the course of HIV disease in about one-half of cases in the U.S., and in higher proportions in developing countries. The differential diagnosis of diarrhea in HIV infection includes the following entities:

* Small intestine: CMV, cryptosporidium, microsporidium, isospora, Mycobacterium avium complex, salmonella species, Campylobacter jejuni, giardia, malabsorption, and drug side effects.
* Large intestine: CMV, cryptosporidium, Mycobacterium avium complex, Shigella flexneri, Clostridium difficile, Campylobacter jejuni, amebiasis,

disseminated histoplasmosis, adenovirus, and rectal Herpes simplex. Kaposi's sarcoma and tuberculosis are believed rarely to cause diarrhea in AIDS.

Diagnostic Work-up of Diarrhea:
-Stain for stool WBC's
-Stool culture for bacteria
-Parasite exam (O&P) on three different specimens
-Testing for Clostridium difficile toxin
-Stain for acid-fast bacteria

If all are negative, the patient should be offered colonoscopy with biopsy to detect CMV, HSV, adenovirus, or mycobacteria. Esophagogastro--duodenoscopy with duodenal biopsy may also be indicated to detect CMV, mycobacteria, or microsporidiosis.

d) Hepatobiliary Infection with CMV (12,20)

CMV has been found to cause several hepatobiliary diseases in AIDS, including hepatitis (fever, right upper quadrant pain, jaundice, tender hepatomegaly, mildly elevated transaminases and alkaline phosphatase), cholangiopathy, and acalculous cholecystitis.

CMV cholangiopathy typically presents with RUQ pain, fever, tender hepatomegaly, markedly elevated alkaline phosphatase, mildly elevated transaminases, and normal bilirubin. Imaging studies (CT or ultrasound) may show ductular abnormalities, and cholangiography may reveal choledochal narrowing and dilation, long choledochal strictures, or papillary stenosis.

The differential diagnosis of AIDS cholangiopathy includes microsporidium and cryptosporidium (which can also cause acalculous cholecystitis).

An isolated elevation in alkaline phosphatase with hepatomegaly can result from Mycobacterium avium complex infection.

e) CMV Polyradiculopathy (4)

History: Diffuse, usually bilateral leg pain and ascending weakness, with plantar and perineal paresthesias and urinary retention, progressing over 3-4 weeks and resulting in inability to walk.

CD4 count is usually <50 T-helper cells per microliter.

Physical Exam: Flaccid paraparesis with decreased or absent deep tendon reflexes over lower extremities. Ascending sensory impairment, less severe than motor deficits. Upper extremities are not affected unless disease is allowed to progress untreated. MRI of the spine may be helpful in ruling out vacuolar myelopathy and lymphoma.

Labs: CSF classically shows neutrophilic pleocytosis (average cell count 450), increased protein (average 274 mg/dl), and decreased glucose (average 30 mg/dl). CMV radiculopathy has been observed to occur in the absence of classic CSF findings, however, and some physicians will begin treatment on the basis of clinical presentation alone, as the disease is progressive and fatal if untreated.

CSF CMV culture is approximately 50% sensitive, but treatment should not be delayed pending results.

Differential Diagnosis of Peripheral Neuropathy:

Peripheral neuropathies (4,13) are frequent complications of HIV infection. Secondary neuropathies may result from vincristine chemotherapy for Kaposi's sarcoma, neurotoxicity from the antivirals ddI and ddC, isoniazid treatment for TB with inadequate pyridoxine intake, or from localized compression in bed-bound patients.

Primary Neuropathies in Patients with HIV:

Chronic demyelinating polyneuropathy (CIDP) occurs early in the course of HIV disease, and may be the first evidence of HIV infection. CIDP is characterized by axonal demyelination, resembles Guillan-Barre syndrome in presentation, and may respond to plasmapheresis.

Distal sensory (symmetric) polyneuropathy (DSPN) usually occurs following other complications of immunodeficiency, presenting with paresthesias of the feet and pain on weight-bearing. Objective findings are few, but deficits of vibratory sensation may develop. DSPN is a stable or slowly progressive condition, and motor involvement is rare. The neuropathic pain may respond to treatment with tricyclic antidepressants (amitriptyline, 25-50 mg po qhs, or nortriptyline, 10-75 mg po qhs). Carbamazepine, starting dose 100-200 mg po bid, may also be effective.

Mononeuropathy multiplex is uncommon. It is a patchy, asymmetrical process, and may have both sensory and motor components. Etiology and optimal therapy are unknown.

Comparison of CMV Polyradiculopathy with the Primary Neuropathies:

	CMV	CIDP	DSPN
Frequency	Rare	rare	common
Setting	advanced AIDS	pre-AIDS	AIDS
Urinary retention	present	absent	absent
Hypoesthesia	saddle+plantar	distal	distal
Arm weakness	late	early	late
Cranial nerves affected	late	early	spared
↓ tendon reflexes	distal	generalized	distal
Ascending spinal sensory level	often	absent	absent
CSF:			
Average cell count	449 (71% N)	6 (3% N)	0
Average glucose	29 mg/dl	55 mg/dl	63 mg/dl
Average protein	247 mg/dl	127 mg/dl	50 mg/dl

f) CMV encephalitis (2,7):

History: Altered mental status, fever and confusion, progressive over days to 1-2 weeks. Seizures may occur.
Physical Exam: Non-specific. CT scan usually unremarkable.
Labs: CSF shows neutrophilic pleocytosis.

    Brain biopsy shows intranuclear inclusions without evidence of other etiologic process.

g) CMV pneumonia:

    CMV is frequently detected in pulmonary secretions and biopsies from AIDS patients, but the role of CMV as a pulmonary pathogen in AIDS is uncertain. It has been shown that isolation of CMV from pulmonary sources at the time of PCP diagnosis does not have an adverse effect on survival (3). CMV detected in the presence of other pulmonary pathogens is therefore not treated.

    A minority (<5%) of AIDS patients with pneumonia, however, present with dry cough, dyspnea, diffuse interstitial infiltrates on chest X-ray, and no pathogenic organisms detectable on transbronchial biopsy or broncho-alveolar lavage. Most of these patients have a non-specific pneumonitis that is self-limited and not due to CMV. However, a minority of these patients do have CMV detectable (as nuclear inclusion bodies or positive culture) in bronchial washings or biopsy. In the setting of clinical deterioration, these patients should be treated for CMV.

3. Treatment of Cytomegalovirus Disease:

Because the differential diagnoses for the varied presentations of CMV are extensive, and because the available treatments are toxic, it is essential that positive diagnosis be made and that alternative diagnoses be ruled out before therapy is undertaken (an exception is CMV radiculopathy, for which therapy should not be delayed if neutrophilic CSF pleocytosis, flaccid paraparesis, and ascending neurological deficits are present). Retinal lesions should be examined by an ophthalmologist experienced in the ocular manifestations of AIDS, and gastrointestinal lesions should be examined and biopsied by an endoscopist.

CMV retinitis can rapidly progress to blindness if not treated. Lesions that are threatening vision by virtue of their location (adjacent to the fovea or optic disc in an eye with functional vision) require immediate treatment. Lesions that are peripheral may be either treated or closely monitored for expansion. Since destroyed retina is not recovered by treatment, there is no indication to treat lesions that have already eliminated functional vision. In this situation, treatment to protect the uninvolved eye, if functional, may be appropriate. Certainly, the uninvolved eye should closely monitored for retinitis.

a) Ganciclovir (7,15)

The nucleoside analog ganciclovir (DHPG) is of proven efficacy in treating CMV retinitis in AIDS. A number of case reports suggest that ganciclovir therapy improves ulcers in CMV esophagitis and mitigates weight loss, fever and diarrhea in CMV colitis, but results of controlled studies are not available. In life-threatening illness such as encephalitis or radiculopathy, it is logical to treat, and recoveries have been reported (4).

The doses used in non-ocular CMV infections are usually the same as those established for retinitis:

The induction dose of ganciclovir is 5 mg/kg IV, infused over 1 hour, bid for 14 to 21 days for retinitis, and 21 to 42 days in the case of GI disease.

Because relapse of retinitis generally occurs 20 to 30 days after cessation of therapy, patients completing induction should be started immediately on maintenance doses of 5 mg/kg qd (or 6 mg/kg 5 days per week) infused over 1 hour. The value of maintenance therapy for GI disease is controversial.

Side Effects of Ganciclovir:

Neutropenia, common and frequently dose-limiting. Absolute neutrophil counts fall below 1000 per microliter in 30-40% of patients, and below 500 in 16%. Neutropenia is exacerbated by other myelosuppressive drugs, including zidovudine (AZT). Neutropenia is reversible with stopping therapy.

<u>Thrombocytopenia</u> is somewhat less common, with platelets falling below 50,000 per microliter in 19% of patients and below 20,000 in 5%.

Less frequent side effects include rash, confusion, GI upset and anemia.

Management of Ganciclovir Therapy:

-The patient is usually hospitalized for at least several days during induction for placement of central line and teaching. Ganciclovir may be administered via peripheral line.

-Monitor CBC with diff and platelets qod during induction and q week during maintenance. Retrospective studies indicate that risk of bacterial infection in HIV patients is not increased when absolute neutrophil count (ANC) is between 500 and 1000 as compared to >1000.

-Ganciclovir should be interrupted for ANC <500 cells/microliter or platelets <10-25,000. Therapy may be restarted when ANC >750 and platelets >25,000.

-Zidovudine (AZT) is generally interrupted when induction therapy is begun, as zidovudine acts synergistically with ganciclovir to suppress bone marrow function, and most patients on this combination develop severe neutropenia. Myelosuppressive chemotherapeutic agents should also be avoided.

-If absolute neutrophil count (ANC) is stable at >750-1000 after two weeks of ganciclovir, it is probably reasonable to restart zidovudine, usually at a reduced dose, and slowly increase the dose with close monitoring of the ANC.

-Serum creatinine should be monitored during induction and every few weeks during maintenance. Dosage should be reduced if creatinine clearance falls below 1.1 ml/kg/min according to the following table:

Ganciclovir Dosage In Renal Insufficiency:

Creatinine Clearance (ml/min/kg)	Dose of Gan-cyclovir (mg/kg)	Dosing Interval
INDUCTION:		
≥1.1	5.00	q 12 hrs
0.7-1.0	2.50	q 12 hrs
0.4-0.6	2.50	q 24 hrs
≤0.3	1.25	q 24 hrs
MAINTENANCE:		
≥1.1	5.000	q day
0.7-1.0	2.500	q day
0.4-0.6	1.250	q day
≤0.3	0.625	q day

Creatinine clearance (Cr Cl) is estimated by the following formula:
For males: Cr Cl = (140 - age)/([creatinine] x 72)
For females: Cr Cl = (140 - age)/([creatinine] x 85)

-Patients with herpes simplex or zoster infections should discontinue acyclovir, as ganciclovir provides coverage of acyclovir-sensitive viruses.

Management of Ganciclovir-induced Neutropenia:

-Intravitreal injections (200 micrograms twice a week) of ganciclovir can control retinitis progression without systemic toxicity. Intravitreal administration can also be achieved by surgical implantation of a slow-releasing device. The emergence of extraocular CMV disease in these patients may limit the usefulness of this approach.

-Myeloid stimulating factors may be used to reverse dose-limiting neutropenia. Both granulocyte-macrophage colony stimulating factor (GM-CSF, 1-8 micrograms/kg/d injected subcutaneously) and granulocyte colony stimulating factor (G-CSF, 300 micrograms subcutaneously three times per week) appear promising in ongoing studies.

-The patient may switch to foscarnet, which appears to have clinical efficacy in patients discontinuing ganciclovir because of myelotoxicity.

b) <u>Foscarnet</u> (5,7,16)

The pyrophosphate analog foscarnet (phosphonoformate) is equivalent in efficacy to ganciclovir in controlling CMV retinitis. While free of the myelotoxicity associated with ganciclovir, foscarnet possesses significant nephrotoxicity.

The induction dose of foscarnet in the setting of normal renal function is 60 mg/kg IV, infused over 1 hour by infusion pump only, tid for 14 to 21 days for retinitis, and 21 to 42 days for gastrointestinal disease.

Because relapse occurs when treatment is discontinued, maintenance therapy is necessary. The initial maintenance dose is 90 to 120 mg/kg/d IV, infused over 2 hours by infusion pump only, with 1 liter NS.

Because foscarnet is both nephrotoxic and renally excreted, the dose must be adjusted frequently (3 times per week during induction and once per week during maintenance). Dosage is based on creatinine clearance and weight, according to the following tables:

<u>INDUCTION THERAPY</u>

Creatinine Clearance (ml/min/kg body wt.)	Dose of Foscarnet (mg/kg/8 hrs)
≥1.6	60.0
1.5	56.5
1.4	53.0
1.3	49.4
1.2	45.9
1.1	42.4
1.0	38.9
0.9	35.3
0.8	31.8
0.7	28.3
0.6	24.8
0.5	21.2
0.4	17.7

Creatinine clearance (Cr Cl) is estimated by the following formula:

For males: Cr Cl = (140 - age)/([creatinine] x 72)

For females: Cr Cl = (140 - age)/([creatinine] x 85)

MAINTENANCE THERAPY

Creatinine Clearance (ml/min/kg body wt.)	Dose of Foscarnet (mg/kg/day)
≥1.4	90
1.2-1.4	78
1.0-1.2	75
0.8-1.0	71
0.6-0.8	63
0.4-0.6	57

Side effects of foscarnet:

Nephrotoxicity is dose-limiting in 10-25% of patients. Increases in serum creatinine are common and acute renal failure has been reported. Serum creatinine should be less than or equal to 2.0 mg/dl to start therapy.

Transient Hypocalcemia, due to the ability of the drug to chelate serum calcium, is the second most common dose-limiting side effect. This is a transient, infusion related, phenomenon, affecting the levels of ionized calcium only.

Arrhythmias, Seizures, probably secondary to acute hypocalcemia.

Hyperphosphatemia, benign and self-limited.

Hypophosphatemia, sometimes severe.

Hypokalemia

Hypomagnesemia

Hypocalcemia, a decrease in total serum calcium.

Anemia, mild.

Penile ulcerations.

Management of Foscarnet Therapy:

-Patients are admitted for induction and placement of an indwelling central venous catheter for chronic therapy. Foscarnet may be given peripherally as a diluted preparation.

-Foscarnet must be administered by an IV infusion pump, as a fatal decrease in the level of ionized calcium may result from accidental rapid infusion.

-Monitor creatinine, Ca, Mg, K, phosphate, and CBC qod during induction and q week during maintenance.

-Manage hypocalcemia, hypokalemia, hypomagnesemia, or hypophosphatemia with oral or IV replacement.

-Avoid concomitant nephrotoxic drugs, such as amphotericin, aminoglycosides, and intravenous pentamidine.

-Keep patient well-hydrated. Loading with NS may reduce risk of nephrotoxicity.
-Discontinue therapy for serum Cr greater than or equal to 2.9 mg/dl. Therapy
may be re-started for serum creatinine <2.0 mg/dl.
-Patients taking acyclovir for herpes simplex or varicella-zoster infections
should discontinue acyclovir, as foscarnet provides coverage of these
viruses. In fact, even acyclovir-resistant HSV and VZV respond to
foscarnet (18,19).

4. Outcome of Cytomegalovirus Infection Therapy:

Over 90% of patients receiving a complete course of induction for CMV
retinitis show an initial response, with regression of lesions visible within 10 to
14 days (15). Visual loss from damaged retina is not reversible. Retinal
detachment may follow treatment.

Interestingly, patients with AIDS and CMV retinitis treated with foscarnet
showed significantly longer survival (mortality rate 46 per 100 patients per year,
median survival 12.6 months) than those patients treated with ganciclovir
(mortality rate 66 per 100 patient-years, median survival 8.5 months) (17). This
benefit may be due to the anti-retroviral activity of foscarnet, or may reflect the
fact that fewer patients on ganciclovir are able to take anti-retroviral drugs
because of neutropenia.

This survival advantage did not apply to patients with even slightly
impaired renal function. Patients with creatinine clearance <1.2 ml/min/kg
(corresponding to a serum creatinine of 1.2 or higher in a 40 year old male) at
initiation of therapy actually had shorter survival on foscarnet.

These survival data suggest that foscarnet is the optimal treatment for
CMV retinitis patients with unimpaired kidney function. Unfortunately, the
unavailability of infusion pumps and home nursing care has made this option
largely inaccessible to San Francisco patients without private insurance. One
option for these patients may be to receive foscarnet induction in the hospital and
switch to ganciclovir for outpatient maintenance.

5. Maintenance Therapy and Follow-up for Cytomegalovirus Disease (7):

Lesions of CMV retinitis recur 20 to 30 days after cessation of therapy.
Maintenance therapy delays, but does not ultimately prevent, recurrence. 30 to
50% of patients will show progression of lesions while on maintenance therapy,
usually after 1 to 4 months.

For this reason, patients should receive regular eye exams during
treatment. Recurrences are usually treated by repeating a 2 week course of

induction and then proceeding with maintenance, usually at a higher dose. (For foscarnet, maintenance doses following second induction are calculated by multiplying the doses in the "Maintenance" table above by a factor of 1.3.)

With chronic ganciclovir therapy, some patients will have progression of lesions and will secrete ganciclovir-resistant CMV in urine. These patients often respond when changed to foscarnet. The benefit of switching to ganciclovir for failure of foscarnet is not known.

Given the non-overlapping toxicities of ganciclovir and foscarnet, combination therapy involving lower doses of both may prove more effective and less toxic than therapy with either alone. Trials of this approach are in progress.

Line infections occur at a rate of 0.3-0.5 infections per 100 catheter days in AIDS patients.

References

1) deSmet MD and RB Nussenbatt. Ocular manifestations of AIDS. JAMA 1991; 226:3019-3022.

2) Jacobson MA and J Mills. Serious CMV disease in the acquired immune deficiency syndrome (AIDS). Annals of Internal Medicine 1988; 108:585-594.

3) Jacobson, MA, et al. Morbidity and mortality of patients with AIDS and first episode PCP unaffected by concomitant pulmonary CMV infection. American Review of Respiratory Disease 1991; 144:6-9.

4) Miller RG, et al. Ganciclovir in the treatment of progressive AIDS-related polyradiculopathy. Neurology 1990; 40:569-574.

5) Palestine AG, et al. A randomized controlled trial of foscarnet in the treatment of CMV retinitis in patients with AIDS. Annals of Internal Medicine 1991; 155:665-673.

6) Wilcox, CM et al. Cytomegalovirus Esophagitis in Patients with AIDS. Annals of Internal Medicine 1990; 113:589-593.

7) Jacobson, MA. Management of CMV retinitis in AIDS. In Mills J, and L Corey, eds. Antiviral Chemotherapy: New Directions for Clinical Applications and Research, vol. 3. 1992, in press.

8) Bach MC, et al. Aphthous ulceration of the GI tract in patients with the acquired immune deficiency syndrome (AIDS). Annals of Internal Medicine 1990; 112: 465-467.

9) Brew JB. Central and peripheral nervous system abnormalities. Medical Clinics of North America (AIDS issue) 1992; 76:63-81.

10) Tamowitz HB, et al. Gastrointestinal Manifestations. Ibid, pp 45-62.

11) Smith PD. Gastrointestinal infections in AIDS. Annals of Internal Medicine 1992; 116:63-77.

12) Cappel MS. Hepatobiliary manifestations of the acquired immune deficiency syndrome. American Journal of Gastroenterology 1991; 86:1-15.

13) Hollander H. Neurologic and psychiatric manifestations of HIV disease. Journal of General Internal Medicine 1991; 6(suppl.):S24-S31.
14) Dietrich DT and M Rahmin. CMV colitis in AIDS: 44 patients and review. Journal of Acquired Immune Deficiency Syndromes 1991; 4(suppl.1):S29-S35.
15) Henderly DE and LM Jampol. Diagnosis and treatment of CMV retinitis. Ibid, pp S6-S10.
16) Jacobson MA and JJ O'Donnell. Approaches to the treatment of cytomegalovirus retinitis: ganciclovir and foscarnet. Ibid, pp S11-S16.
17) Mortality of patients with the acquired immune deficiency syndrome treated with either foscarnet or ganciclovir for cytomegalovirus retinitis. Studies of Ocular Complications of AIDS Research Group, in collaboration with the AIDS clinical Trials Group. NEJM 1992, 326:213-220.
18) Safrin, S, et al. A controlled trial comparing foscarnet with vidarabine for acyclovir-resistant mucocutaneous herpes simplex in the acquired immune deficiency syndrome. NEJM 1991; 325:551-555.
19) Safrin, S et al. Foscarnet therapy in five patients with AIDS and acyclovir--resistant varicella-zoster virus infection. Annals of Internal Medicine 1991; 115:19-21.
20) Chan MF and SL Friedman. CMV and the gastrointestinal system. AIDSFILE 1992; 6:1-2.
21) Cochereau-Massin I, et al. Ocular toxoplasmosis in HIV-infected patients. American Journal of Ophthalmology 1992; 114:130-135.
22) Wilcox CM and DA Schwartz. A pilot study of oral corticosteroid therapy for idiopathic esophageal ulcerations associated with HIV infection. Am J Medicine 1992; 93:131-134.
23) Ryan J, et al. Thalidomide to treat esophageal ulcers in AIDS. NEJM 1992; 327:208-209.

Systemic mycoses: Histoplasma Capsulatum & Coccidioides

I. Histoplasmosis (1,2,4)

Introduction

Histoplasma capsulatum, a soil-dwelling fungus endemic to the Mississippi, Ohio, and St. Lawrence river valleys and the Caribbean, including southern Mexico, causes a systemic, debilitating disease in AIDS patients. Affected tissues may include the lungs, bone marrow, liver, spleen, lymph nodes, skin, and, rarely, the CNS. Disseminated histoplasmosis in AIDS patients is probably due to exogenous exposure, although reactivation has not been excluded. Histoplasmosis accounted for 1% of initial AIDS diagnoses reported in the U.S. in 1990.

Presentation

History: Fever and weight loss, often over weeks or months, occur in over 90% of affected patients. Cough or dyspnea of 1-2 months duration is often noted in those patients with chest x-ray abnormalities, but pulmonary symptoms are often absent in patients with normal chest X-rays. Neurologic, gastrointestinal, or dermatologic complaints are each present in fewer than 20%.

History of travel to endemic areas, especially with activities associated with exposure to aerosols of soil or bird feces (such as excavation, construction, or caving), may raise suspicion of histoplasmosis.

CD4 counts have not been well studied in histoplasmosis, but most patients probably have T-helper counts of <100 cells per microliter.

Physical Exam: Fever is usually present. Lymphadenopathy is common. Hepatomegaly or splenomegaly is found in 10-20%. Papular or pustular skin lesions have been reported.

Approximately 12% will present with a sepsis-like syndrome of hypotension, respiratory insufficiency and renal or hepatic failure. Prognosis is poor in these patients.

Chest X-rays: Diffuse interstitial or reticulonodular infiltrates are present in about one-third of affected patients. Focal infiltrate is present in 10%. Hilar and mediastinal adenopathy with calcified granulomata, the hallmarks of pulmonary histoplasmosis in immunocompetent patients, are present in fewer than 5% of affected AIDS patients. Chest X-ray is normal in approximately 40%.

Labs: CBC shows anemia, leukocytopenia, and thrombocytopenia in about 30%, probably due to bone marrow involvement.

Peripheral blood buffy coat (silver or PAS stain) is 40% sensitive.

Blood cultures are about 90% sensitive.

<u>Bone marrow biopsy</u> stain is 40% sensitive; stain and culture together are 90% sensitive.

<u>Biopsy</u> of enlarged lymph nodes or skin lesions may be diagnostic.

<u>Broncho-alveolar lavage or transbronchial biopsy</u> for diffuse pulmonary infiltrates is frequently diagnostic

<u>Skin testing and serology</u> are not useful, as patients are frequently anergic, and positive results do not establish cause of current illness.

<u>Radioimmunoassay</u> for histoplasma polysaccharide antigen in urine, blood, or CSF is currently in development.

Treatment of Histoplasmosis:

Amphotericin B, 0.5-0.8 mg/kg/d IV to a total dose of 15 mg/kg.

Amphotericin administration and side effects see page 44 for more information. Doses should be increased to the therapeutic dose of 0.5-0.8 mg/kg/d as rapidly as tolerated.

Itraconazole (Sporanox) 300 mg po bid for three days, followed by 200 mg po bid for 12 weeks is currently in clinical trials (ACTG 120). Fluconazole, 400 mg po bid, may also be effective.

Ketoconazole, while sometimes successful in immunocompetent patients with histoplasmosis, is generally unsatisfactory in AIDS patients.

Outcome of Histoplasmosis Therapy:

80% of patients with disseminated histoplasmosis respond to amphotericin B, with lysis of fever by 7 days in about 70%. Prognosis is worse in patients presenting with CNS involvement or sepsis.

Suppressive Therapy and Follow-up:

Relapse occurs frequently after therapy is discontinued. Chronic suppressive therapy with amphotericin B, 1.0 mg/kg q week, prevents relapse within one year in 80-90% of patients.

Anecdotal reports suggest a role for fluconazole (400 mg po qd) in chronic suppressive therapy following initial treatment with 15 mg/kg (total dose) amphotericin. Itraconazole maintenance (200 mg po bid) is currently under study (ACTG 084).

II. Coccidioides Immitis (1,2,3)

Introduction:

The fungus Coccidioides immitis is found in warm, dry soil and is endemic to the southwestern U.S., especially Arizona and the San Joaquin valley of California, as well as arid regions of Mexico and Central and South America. In AIDS patients, coccidioides causes severe pneumonia, with or without extra-- thoracic dissemination that may involve the meninges, joints, skin, liver or lymph nodes. It is uncertain whether disease in AIDS patients results from new exposure or reactivation.

Coccidioidomycosis accounted for 0.25% of initial AIDS diagnoses in the U.S. in 1990.

Presentation:

History: Fever, night sweats, and weight loss are common. Cough and shortness of breath are present in about half of affected patients. Meningitis may manifest as progressive lethargy with fever. History of travel to endemic areas should be elicited.

CD4 count is usually <500 (average 150) in 90% of affected AIDS patients.

Physical Exam: Physical exam is non-specific and may include fever, cachexia, or pulmonary findings.

Chest X-ray: Normal on presentation in about two-thirds of AIDS patients with coccidioidomycosis.
Diffuse infiltrates of a discretely nodular appearance are seen in about half of patients with abnormal x-rays, and focal infiltrates are seen in about one-third. Cavities and intrathoracic adenopathy have also been observed.

Labs: Broncho-alveolar lavage or transbronchial biopsy with histologic exam and fungal culture have a high diagnostic yield in patients with respiratory signs and symptoms.
Blood cultures for fungus are positive in only 12% of patients with lung involvement.
Coccidioides serologies are about 90% sensitive, but may be negative in the most severely immunocompromised patients. Specificity is uncertain.
CSF in patients with coccidioidal meningitis usually shows a lymphocytic pleocytosis of >50 cells per microliter (i.e., more cells than usually seen in cryptococcal meningitis), elevated protein, and depressed glucose. Examination of CSF may reveal the organism. CSF culture is 60% sensitive.
Lymph node biopsy, with stain and culture, may be diagnostic.

Skin testing is not useful, being <20% sensitive.

Treatment of Coccidioides Infection:

Treatment consists of amphotericin B, 0.5 to 0.8 mg/kg/d to a total dose of 2 to 2.5 g.

Administration and side effects of amphotericin B see page 44 for more information. Doses should be increased to the therapeutic dose of 0.5-0.8 mg/kg/d as rapidly as tolerated.

Trials of fluconazole (400 mg qd) and itraconazole appear encouraging in the setting of coccidioidal meningitis. As CSF penetration of amphotericin B may be inadequate, intrathecal therapy may be combined with systemic therapy in patients with coccidioidal meningitis.

Outcome of Coccidioides Therapy:

Prognosis of diffuse pulmonary involvement is poor; 70% of patients with HIV infection and reticulonodular pulmonary coccidioides die despite the use of amphotericin B. Median survival is one month. CNS involvement is also associated with a very poor prognosis.

Suppressive Therapy and Follow-up:

Lifelong suppressive therapy is required, as even brief cessation of therapy may result in relapse. The optimal regimen is under investigation. Currently, maintenance therapy consists of either fluconazole, 200 mg po bid, or amphotericin B, 1 mg/kg once or twice per week. Maintenance therapy with ketoconazole is not recommended because of a reportedly high relapse rate (J.D. Stansell, personal communication).

References

1) Terrell CL and CE Hughes. Antifungal agents used for deep-seated mycotic infections. Mayo Clinic Proceedings 1992; 67:69-91.
2) Gagliani JN and Ampel NM. Coccidoides in HIV patients. Journal of Infectious Diseases 1990; 162:1165-1169.
3) Stansell JD. Disseminated histoplasmosis and coccidioidomycosis infections in HIV-infected patients. AIDSFILE 1991; 5:2-5.
4) Wheat IJ, et al. Disseminated histoplasmosis in the acquired immune deficinecy syndrome: clinical findings, diagnosis and treatment, and review of the literature. Medicine 1990; 69:361-374.

Mycobacterium Avium Complex

1. Introduction

Infection with the Mycobacterium avium complex (MAC, also called MAI), consisting of the closely related species M. avium and M. intracellulare, causes a progressive, disseminated illness in patients with AIDS involving the blood, bone marrow, liver, spleen, lungs, and GI tract, and, less commonly, the CNS, pelvic viscera, and skin. Disseminated MAC infection occurs in 15-25% of AIDS patients in the U.S., usually late in the course of HIV infection.

Disease appears to be due to primary acquisition rather than reactivation, with dissemination originating from focal pulmonary or gastrointestinal sites. MAC is not pathogenic in the non-immunocompromised host, although asymptomatic, non-disseminating colonization of the respiratory or GI tract may occur.

There is no particular region or risk group associated with MAC infection in the U.S. The organisms are ubiquitous in food, water, and soil, making avoidance of exposure unfeasible.

2. Presentation

History: The great majority of patients experience persistent fever (with or without night sweats), weight loss, and malaise. Chronic diarrhea, nausea, abdominal pain, and, infrequently, symptoms of biliary obstruction may also be present. Weight loss and diarrhea have both been found to be significantly associated with isolation of MAC from blood cultures (4). Prominent pulmonary symptoms are unusual. Asymptomatic disseminated MAC infection is not observed.

Infection is very rare in patients with CD4 count >100. At San Francisco General Hospital, 96-98% of patients with disseminated MAC have <50 CD4 cells per microliter (J.D. Stansell, unpublished data.) MAC organisms are detectable in blood cultures in about 36% of HIV-infected patients with CD4 counts <100 (2). A recent study (8) found that 21% of patients surviving 1 year after AIDS diagnosis developed MAC bacteremia; this percentage doubled after the second year. It was also observed that MAC bacteremia developed in 39% of patients surviving 1 year after their CD4 count fell to < 10 cells per microliter.

Physical Exam: Non specific. Fever and cachexia are common. Hepatospleno-megaly is sometimes observed.

Labs: Anemia (Hct <26) is significantly associated with positive blood cultures for MAC, as is elevation of alkaline phosphatase to more than 3 times normal (4). Blood culture X 2 provides up to 98% sensitivity. Bone marrow, lymph nodes, and bowel wall biopsy and culture are also relatively sensitive. Stool, sputum, and broncho-alveolar lavage fluid are somewhat less sensitive (average 60% for each site). MAC is isolated from urine in 43% and from CSF in about 11% of patients. The presence of MAC in non-sterile body sites is suggestive, but not diagnostic, of disseminated disease, as about one-third of colonized AIDS patients develop dissemination within 5 months (6).

The radiometric Bactec system, if available, detects growth in 6-12 days. Culture on Loewenstein-Jensen agar takes 2-3 weeks or longer.

Chest X-ray: Pneumonia occurs in only about 4% of patients with disseminated MAC. Chest X-ray is non-specific. Slowly progressive nodular densities are frequently observed, but infiltrates may also be diffuse or patchy. Intrathoracic adenopathy may be present. Cavities, effusion and miliary pattern are uncommon. Chest X-ray may be normal.

CT scan: Abdominal CT scan may reveal marked hepatosplenomegaly, diffuse jejunal wall thickening, or large retroperitoneal or mesenteric lymph nodes. In MAC infection, enlarged nodes tend to be of homogeneous soft tissue density. Central low attenuation, characteristic of caseation necrosis, is more suggestive of tuberculosis (6).

3. Treatment of Mycobacterium Avium Complex:

There is no definitive treatment for infection with MAC, and no treatment has been shown to prolong survival. However, several trials indicate that reduction of colony counts on blood culture by antimicrobial therapy is associated with improvement of symptoms in most patients (1). Many clinicians at feel that improvement in quality of life is sufficient to justify treatment despite the lack of survival data.

Significant suppression of bacteremia with improvement of fever and night sweats and increased feeling of well-being has been reported with the following oral regimen (1):

Rifampin, 10 mg/kg (max. 600 mg) per day
Ethambutol, 15-25 mg/kg (max 1000 mg) per day
Clofazamine, 100 mg per day
Ciprofloxacin, 500-750 mg bid.

Nausea, vomiting, diarrhea, and abdominal pain were commonly observed with this regimen, and weight loss was not improved. In addition, side effects associated with the individual drugs include the following (2):

Rifampin: Rash, nausea, vomiting, increased liver enzymes, alterations in serum drug levels (fluconazole level decreases by 25%, ketoconazole by 80%, dapsone by up to 90%)

    <u>Ethambutol</u>: Decreased visual acuity (optic neuritis), abdominal pain

    <u>Clofazamine</u>: Skin darkening and dryness, rash, abdominal pain, nausea and vomiting

    <u>Ciprofloxacin</u>: Nausea, vomiting, abdominal pain, rash, headache, seizures.

Clarithromycin (Biaxin), a recently licensed macrolide antibiotic, has efficacy against a high percentage of MAC isolates, and relatively low toxicity. Clarithromycin has been shown in a placebo-controlled crossover study to reduce MAC colony counts in AIDS patients (7). If used for MAC, clarithromycin should be given in combination with other antibiotics, as emergence of resistant strains occurs rapidly when single-drug therapy is used. One regimen used at SFGH (J.D. Stansell, personal communication, 1992) consists of:

Clarithromycin, 1.0 gm po bid (If poorly tolerated, 0.5 gm bid may be used.)
Ethambutol, 25 mg/kg po qd
Ciprofloxacin, 500-750 mg po bid.

Because of the high cost of this regimen, clofazamine, 100 mg po qd, is often substituted for ciprofloxacin.

Common side effects of clarithromycin include nausea, vomiting, and a metallic taste.

The aminoglycoside Amikacin, 10 mg/kg IV qd, has also been included in anti-MAC regimens, and it has been recommended as adjunctive therapy in patients who do not respond after 4-6 weeks of oral treatment alone (2). However, ototoxicity is a frequent side effect when amikacin is used for more than 8 weeks, and may not be detected early enough to prevent irreversible hearing loss. Nephrotoxicity is also common.

The possibility of tuberculosis should be considered when acid-fast bacilli are detected in a specimen from a patient with HIV infection. If tuberculosis is suspected, anti-Tb therapy should always be instituted until culture results are available, as the consequences of untreated Tb are much more serious than those of MAC infection.

4. Outcome of Mycobacterium Avium Complex Therapy:

Fever, night sweats, and malaise may respond to therapy within 2 to 8 weeks. Diarrhea, weight loss, and elevated alkaline phosphatase resolve less frequently, and anemia seldom responds (2).

Patients with disseminated MAC infection have significantly shortened survival. One study, controlled for CD4 count and anti-retroviral therapy, found a median survival of 4.1 months in patients with disseminated MAC, versus 11.1 months in non-MAC infected patients (5). Another series at SFGH found similar survivals (3.5 months versus 9.5 months) (3). Severe weight loss and malnutrition probably contribute to the demise of these patients. No controlled studies evaluating the effect of treatment for MAC on survival are available.

6. Suppressive Therapy and Follow-up:

Dramatic rebound in blood culture colony counts occurs in patients who discontinue therapy (1). If clinical response occurs, suppressive therapy should probably be continued for life.

7. Prophylaxis

The status of chemoprophylaxis against MAC infection is not established. Prophylaxis against disseminated MAC may be appropriate for patients with fewer than 100 CD4 cells or for those with demonstrated colonization. The experimental drug rifabutin, 300 mg qd, has been shown to delay the development of MAC bacteremia, but has shown no effect on survival (9). Pending licensure, the drug is available from Adria Laboratories (800-552-7228) for treatment of HIV-infected patients with CD4 counts of 200 or less. The macrolides azithromycin and clarithromycin are also being studied.

References

1) Kemper CA, et al. Treatment of Mycobacterium avium complex bacteremia in AIDS with a four drug oral regimen. Annals of Internal Medicine 1992; 164: 994-998.
2) Horsburgh CR, Jr. Mycobacterium avium complex in the acquired immune deficiency syndrome. NEJM 1991; 324:1332-1339.
3) Jacobson MA, et al. Natural history of disseminated Mycobacterium avium complex infection in AIDS. Journal of Infectious Diseases 1991; 164:994-998.
4) Havlik JA, Jr., et al. Disseminated Mycobacterium avium complex infection: clinical, identification, and epidemiologic trends. Journal of Infectious diseases 1992; 165:577-580.
5) Horsburgh CR, Jr., et al. Survival of patients with AIDS and disseminated Mycobacterium avium infection with and without antimicrobial chemotherapy. American Review of Respiratory Disease 1991; 144:557-559.
6) Pitchenik AE, and D Fertel. Medical management of AIDS patients. Tuberculous and non-tuberculous mycobacterial disease. Medical Clinics of North America 1992; 76:121-171.
7) Dautzenberg B, et al. Activity of clarithromycin against Mycobacterium avium infection in patients with the acquired immune deficiency syndrome. American Review of Respiratory Disease 1991; 144:564-569.
8) Nightingale SD, et al. Incidence of Mycobacterium avium-intracellulare

complex bacteremia in HIV-positive patients. Journal of Infectious Diseases 1992; 165:1082-1085.

9) Cameron WD, et al. Rifabutin therapy for the prevention of M. avium complex bacteremia in patients with AIDS and CD4 < 200. Abstr. WeB 1055, VIII Intl. Conf. on AIDS, Amsterdam 1992.

Co-morbid Infections

The following illnesses may affect non-immunocompromised patients, but raise particular management issues in the setting of HIV infection.

Tuberculosis

Epidemiology and Presentation:

HIV infection greatly increases the chance of developing TB in persons infected with Mycobacterium tuberculosis (1). Furthermore, HIV-infected persons exposed to TB are likely to have rapidly progressive primary disease rather than subclinical infection (5). Extrapulmonary dissemination occurs in the majority of patients with full-blown AIDS and pulmonary TB, and in a large minority of those with less advanced HIV infection (3). M. tb. is isolated from the CSF in 10% of patients with HIV and tuberculosis. (For a discussion of TB meningitis, see "Differential diagnosis of CSF abnormalities," page 41.)

Clinical and radiographic presentation of TB in patients with otherwise asymptomatic HIV infection tends to be similar to presentation in HIV-negative patients. In more advanced HIV infection, intrathoracic lymphadenopathy and/or diffuse infiltrates may be observed (8).

Respiratory precautions:

Transmission of M. tb to health care workers is not unusual (6). Respiratory precautions must be taken with coughing patients until TB has been ruled out, either by establishing another diagnosis that fully explains pulmonary symptoms and x-ray appearance, or by negative AFB staining of three consecutive sputum samples.

Purified Protein Derivative (PPD) Evaluation:

PPD should be placed subcutaneously, using 5 Tuberculin Units, as early as possible in patients with HIV or at high risk of HIV infection. Patients reacting with 5 mm of induration (as opposed to the usual 10 mm) are considered exposed, as are those who report positive skin test in the past. If active infection is excluded by chest X-ray, exposed patients should receive INH, 5 mg/kg/d (maximum dose 300 mg qd), plus pyridoxine, 25-50 mg qd, for at least 12 months (7). Prophylaxis is also appropriate for anergic patients (those with negative controls as well as negative PPD) at high risk of exposure by history or social situation (10).

PPD testing is of limited use in diagnosing active disease in patients with HIV infection. 70% of those who develop TB prior to AIDS diagnosis have a positive skin test, but **only 33% of those who develop TB following a diagnosis of AIDS will have a positive PPD.**

Treatment of Tuberculosis:

Therapy for TB in the setting of HIV disease has been described (3,4), and the antituberculous drugs available in the US have been recently reviewed (8,9). The standard regimen consists of three or four drugs, each given as a single daily dose:

Isoniazid (INH), 5 mg/kg/d po (maximum dose 300 mg/d) +
Rifampin, 10 mg/kg/d po or IV (maximum dose 600 mg/d)+
Pyrazinamide (PZA), 15-25 mg/kg/d po;
Ethambutol, 15-25 mg/kg/d po is added if INH resistance is suspected, or in the case of disseminated or CNS infection.

All three (or four) drugs should be given for at least 2 months. INH and rifampin should then be continued for at least 9 months, or for 6 months after conversion of TB cultures to negative, whichever is longer. Pyridoxine (vitamin B6), 25-50 mg qd, should be given to patients receiving INH. Rifampin reduces the serum concentrations of several drugs, including fluconazole. Ketoconazole reduces the absorption of rifampin, and this interaction may lead to TB treatment failure (11).

90% of drug-resistant cases of TB in the US in recent years have occurred in HIV-infected patients (1), requiring alternative treatment regimens. If drug-resistant disease or exposure is suspected, a TB specialist should be consulted. The possibility of transmission of these organisms to other patients and to health care workers highlights the necessity of respiratory precautions.

Suggested reading

1) Snider DE, Jr and NL Roper. The new tuberculosis. NEJM 1992; 326:703-705.
2) Berenguer J, et al. Tuberculous meningitis in patients infected with the human immunodeficiency virus. NEJM 1992; 326:668-672.
3) Barnes PF, et al. Tuberculosis in patients with human immunodeficiency virus infection. NEJM 1991; 324:1644-1650.
4) Small PM, et al. Treatment of tuberculosis in patients with advanced human immunodeficiency virus infection. NEJM 1991; 324:289-294.
5) Daley CL, et al. An outbreak of tuberculosis with accelerated progression among persons infected with the human immunodeficiency virus. An analysis uding restriction-fragment-length-polymorphisms. NEJM 1992; 326:231-235.
6) Pierce JR, Jr., et al. Transmission of tuberculosis to hospital workers by a

patient with AIDS. Chest 1992; 101:581-582.
7) White DA and MK Zaman. Medical management of AIDS patients: Pulmonary disease. Medical Clinics of North America 1992; 45:163-168.
8) Van Scoy RE and CJ Wilkowske. Antituberculous agents. Mayo Clinic Proceedings 1992; 67:179-187.
9) The Medical Letter on Drugs and Therapeutics. Drugs for Tuberculosis. 1992; 34:10-12.
10) Selwyn PA, et al. High risk of active tuberculosis in HIV-infected drug users with cutaneous anergy. JAMA 1992; 268:504-509.
11) Engelhard D, et al. Interaction of ketoconazole with rifampin and isoniazid. NEJM 1984; 311:1681-1683.

Syphilis

There is anecdotal evidence that syphilis may pursue a more aggressive course in HIV-infected patients, and that response to established treatment regimens may be delayed or incomplete (1). At this time, appropriate treatment for all stages of syphilis in HIV-infected individuals remains controversial.

Late Latent versus Neurosyphilis:

While clinicians should always consider the possibility of neurosyphilis in HIV-infected patients with altered mental status or neurologic abnormalities, diagnosis is complicated by the fact that CSF abnormalities frequently found in HIV infection (lymphocytic pleocytosis, elevated protein, oligoclonal bands) mimic those of neurosyphilis. While a positive CSF-VDRL is believed to be specific for neurosyphilis, false negative CSF serologies are not unusual in the setting of HIV infection. For these reasons, the use of lumbar puncture for the sole purpose of diagnosing neurosyphilis in AIDS patients is controversial (2).

All patients with HIV infection should have a serum VDRL (or RPR). If this screening test is positive, a confirmatory serum treponemal test (FTA-ABS or MHATP) should be done. If treponemal infection is confirmed and serologies have been positive for longer than one year (or for unknown duration), the patient should probably be offered lumbar puncture for CSF cell count and CSF-VDRL, especially if abnormal neuropsychiatric signs are present. (Any HIV-infected patient undergoing lumbar puncture for disease of other suspected etiology should have a CSF-VDRL sent as well.)

If the CSF is normal, the patient should be treated for late latent syphilis (Benzathine penicillin, 2.4 million U IM q week for three weeks). If the CSF VDRL is positive, the patient must be treated for neurosyphilis (Aqueous penicillin G, 2-4 million U IV q 4 hrs for 10 days; or procaine penicillin, 2.4 million U IM qd, plus probenecid, 500 mg po qd, for 10 days; either regimen should be followed by benzathine penicillin, 2.4 million units IM q week for three weeks) (3).

Ceftriaxone, 1 gram IM qd for 10 days, is currently being investigated as treatment for neurosyphilis.

If the CSF-VDRL is negative but the CSF shows a lymphocytic pleocytosis, it is not unreasonable for the HIV-infected patient with positive serum VDRL and FTA-ABS to receive full treatment for neurosyphilis, especially if neuropsychiatric abnormalities are present.

Early Syphilis:

CDC recommendations for treatment of primary or secondary syphilis, or latent syphilis of less than one year's duration, are the same as for non-HIV infected patients (benzathine penicillin, 2.4 million U IM x 1). Some authorities, however, recommend three doses at weekly intervals because of the anecdotal likelihood of relapse to neurosyphilis in HIV-infected patients receiving only a single injection (1).

Suggested reading
1) Musher DM, et al. Effect of human immunodeficiency virus infection on the course of neurosyphilis and on the response to treatment. Annals of Internal Medicine 1990; 113:872-881.
2) Cooke M, et al. Controversies in the management of HIV-related illnesses. Journal of General Internal Medicine 1991; 6(1 suppl.):S46-S55.
3) The Medical Letter on Drugs and Therapeutics. Drugs for AIDS and Associated Infections. 1991; 33:95-102.
4) Hook EW. Syphilis and HIV infection. Journal of Infectious Diseases 1989; 160:530-534.
5) Tramont C. Controversies regarding the natural history and treatment of syphilis in HIV disease. In P Volberding and M Jacobson, eds. AIDS Clinical Review 1991. New York. Marcel Dekker. pp 97-107.

Candidiasis

The yeast Candida albicans is an extremely common pathogen in HIV--infected patients. While candidemia with dissemination may occur, especially as a vascular catheter-related infection, candidiasis usually occurs in the mouth, esophagus, or vagina.

a)   Oral candidiasis

Oral candidiasis (thrush) occurs in more than half of HIV-infected patients with CD4 counts <200. It is not unusual in patients with >500 CD4 cells and is therefore often the first sign of HIV infection. Oral candidiasis presents as white, friable plaques on the buccal mucosa, tongue (especially the sides of the posterior portion) or palate. Diagnosis may be made by KOH smear. Culture is rarely necessary. The differential diagnosis includes hairy leukoplakia and human papilloma virus infection.

Treatment of Oral Candidiasis:

<u>Clotrimazole</u> (Mycelex) troches, 10 mg dissolved in mouth over 15-30 minutes, 3-5 times a day for 2 weeks. Side effects include hepatotoxicity and lower abdominal cramps.

<u>Nystatin (Mycostatin)</u>: oral pastilles (200,000 units), one to two dissolved slowly in mouth five times a day; or vaginal tablets (100,000 U), dissolved slowly in mouth three times a day. Side effects include transient nausea, vomiting or diarrhea.

<u>Ketoconazole</u> (Nizoral), 200 mg po qd for two weeks. Ketoconazole requires an acidic gastric pH to be absorbed, and should not be taken with H-2 blockers or antacids, or within two hours of the antiviral dideoxyinosine (ddl), which contains an alkaline buffer. Side effects include anorexia, nausea, vomiting, potentially serious hepatotoxicity, and inhibition of steroid (testosterone, estradiol, cortisol, mineralocorticoid) synthesis. Ketoconazole should not be used in the setting of liver disease, and should be discontinued if increases in liver enzymes occur. Ketoconazole may decrease serum levels of rifampin, leading to TB treatment failure. Serious cardiac arrhythmias have occurred when ketoconazole is taken concurrently with the antihistamine, terfenadine (Seldane) (2).

<u>Fluconazole</u> (Diflucan), 50-100 mg po qd. More expensive than ketoconazole, but associated with less toxicity. More effective and associated with less frequent relapse than clotrimazole (6). Occasional side effects include nausea, headache, skin rash, abdominal pain, vomiting, and diarrhea. Elevation in liver transaminases may also occur.

b)   <u>Candida Esophagitis</u>:

Candidiasis of the esophagus accounts for approximately 15% of new AIDS diagnoses in the U.S., and is now the second most common AIDS-defining opportunistic infection in the U.S., after PCP (5). The disease usually presents as difficulty swallowing, and patients commonly complain that food is "sticking." Pain on swallowing suggests another cause (also see CMV esophagitis, page 48) Oral thrush is usually, but not always, present.

If dysphagia alone is present, empiric treatment with ketoconazole (200-400 mg po qd; see above for precautions) or fluconazole (100-200 mg po qd) may be attempted. Although more expensive, fluconazole provides a higher rate of clinical and endoscopic cure than does ketoconazole (7). If improvement occurs, therapy should be continued for 14-21 days. Daily ketoconazole (200 mg) or fluconazole (100 mg) maintenance may then be required to prevent relapse. If no improvement occurs after 7-10 days of empiric therapy, endoscopy should be offered.

c) <u>Candida Vaginitis</u>:

Candida vaginitis is common early in the course of HIV infection, and may be related to immunosuppression. A prospective study of 66 women infected with HIV (3) showed a hierarchy of affected sites associated with decreasing CD4 counts:

Mean CD4 Count	Infection
750	None
510	Vaginal
230	Oropharyngeal
30	Esophageal

Candida vaginitis may be treated with commercially available creams or tablets (clotrimazole, nystatin, or miconazole). Ketoconazole, 200 mg po qd for 10 days (see above for precautions), may be used for severe disease. Cures have been reported with fluconazole, 400 mg po as a single dose.

<u>Suggested reading</u>
1) Greenspan D. The management of fungal diseases of the mouth in HIV infection. AIDSFILE 1991; 5:5-7.
2) The Medical Letter on Drugs and Therapeutics. Safety of terfenadine and astemizole. 1992; 34:9-10.
3) Iman N, et al. Hierarchical pattern of mucosal candida infection in HIV seropositive women. American Journal of Medicine 1990; 89:142-146.
4) Cello JP. AIDS-associated gastrointestinal disease. In MA Sande and PA Volberding, eds. <u>The Medical Management of AIDS, 2nd ed</u>. Saunders. 1990.
5) Farizo KM, et al. Spectrum of disease in persons with human immunodeficiency virus infection in the United States. JAMA 1992; 267:1798-1805.
6) Koletar SL et al. Comparison of oral fluconazole and clotrimazole troches as a treatment for oral candidiasis in patients in patients infected with human immunodeficiency virus. Antimicrobial agents and Chemotherapy 1990; 34:2267-2268.
7) Laine L, et al. Fluconazole compared with ketoconazole for the treatment of candida esophagitis in AIDS: a randomized trial. Annals of Internal Medicine 1992; 117:655-660.

Intestinal Parasites

The intestinal protozoan Cryptosporidium (4) affects 3-4% of AIDS patients in the US (probably > 50% in Africa), causing an enteritis characterized by severe watery diarrhea, cramping abdominal pain, anorexia, weight loss, and malaise. Nausea, vomiting, fever, and myalgias are also observed. Cryptosporidium may also infect the bile ducts and gall bladder, causing symptoms of cholecystitis or cholangitis. Rarely, the organism causes an interstitial pneumonia resembling PCP.

In immunocompetent hosts, and in HIV-infected patients with >200 CD4 cells, symptoms resolve spontaneously and infection is usually cleared within 4 weeks. However, 87% of HIV-infected patients with CD4 count <140 infected with Cryptosporidium will develop persistent disease (1). In these patients, diarrhea is voluminous (1 to 20 liters per day), malaise is debilitating, and wasting and pain may be severe.

Diagnosis is usually made by stool samples (at least 3) examined for ova and parasites. Excretion may be intermittent.

Treatment is primarily palliative, as no antimicrobial agent has been particularly effective. Antispasmodics, antidiarrheals, and antiemetics should be used liberally, with fluid and electrolyte replacement as needed. In addition to opiate derivatives (including tincture of opium), octreotide (Sandostatin), 50-500 micrograms sub-Q tid, may be effective in improving diarrhea (2).

Among antiparasitic agents, paromomycin (Humatin), 566C80 (Atovaquone), and spiramycin have all been disappointing. Hyperimmune bovine colostrum (3) is currently in clinical trials.

Other intestinal protozoan pathogens in AIDS include Isospora belli (4) and microsporidia (Enterocytozoon bieneusi) (5). Both cause severe diarrhea. Isospora usually responds to TMP/SMX, 2 double-strength tablets bid for 2-4 weeks, followed by chronic suppression (TMP/SMX, 1 DS tablet qod).

There is no proven therapy for microsporidium. Metronidazole has been reported to give clinical improvement in some cases, but does not eradicate the parasite. Albendazole, 400 mg bid for 4-6 weeks, appears promising. Symptoms should be treated as in cryptosporidiosis.

<u>Suggested reading</u>

1) Flanigan T., et al. Cryptosporidium infection and CD4 counts. Annals of Internal Medicine 1992; 116:840-842.

2) Cello JP, et al. Effect of octreotide on refractory AIDS-associated diarrhea. Annals of Internal Medicine 1991; 155:705-710.

3) Ungar, BLP, et al. Gastroenterology 1990; 98:486-489.

4) Soave R and WD Johnson, Jr. AIDS commentary: Cryptosporidium and Isospora belli infections. Journal of Infectious Diseases 1988; 157:225-229.

5) Eeftinck Schattenkirk JK, et al. Clinical significance of small intestinal microsporidiosis in HIV-1 infected individuals. Lancet 1991; 337:895-898.

Herpes Viruses

Herpes simplex virus (HSV) types I and II and varicella-zoster virus (VZV) commonly present as reactivated infection in HIV-infected individuals, and may produce more extensive tissue damage than is seen in non-immunocompromised persons. In addition, the frequency and severity of recurrences, and the duration of symptoms tend to be greater in the setting of HIV infection.

Herpes simplex:

HSV may present as orolabial, anorectal, genital or other mucocutaneous lesions, usually accompanied by severe local pain. The majority of homosexual men with AIDS have been previously infected with HSV. Perianal lesions may be confused with decubiti, and should be cultured if the diagnosis is uncertain. True proctitis may present with severe anorectal pain, tenesmus, or sacral radiculopathy, including impotence or neurogenic bladder. Cultures may be necessary to distinguish herpes from gonococcal proctitis (2). Visceral or disseminated infections, including herpes esophagitis (see CMV esophagitis, page 48) and herpes meningoencephalitis are also seen in HIV-infected patients.

Treatment (3,4) of Primary or Recurrent Mucocutaneous HSV in HIV-infected Patients:

Acyclovir (Zovirax), 200-400 mg po 5 times per day for 7-14 days. Duration of treatment depends on clinical response. In severe cases, acyclovir may also be given intravenously (5 mg/kg IV, infused over 1 hr, q 8 hrs.). In the case of visceral organ involvement (eye, esophagus) or neurologic complication (encephalitis, atonic bladder), higher IV doses (10 mg/kg IV, infused over 1 hr, q 8 hrs) may be given.

Many patients will develop recurrences shortly after antiviral therapy is discontinued. Suppressive therapy consists of acyclovir, 400 mg po bid.

Side effects of oral acyclovir include gastrointestinal disturbances and headache. IV acyclovir can cause renal damage; patients should be well hydrated and creatinine should be monitored. IV and, rarely, oral acyclovir may cause CNS side effects, including confusion, tremor, delirium, seizures, and coma. As acyclovir is excreted by the kidney, dosage adjustment is recommended for patients with impaired renal function.

Lesions that do not respond to treatment should be cultured for acyclovir resistance. Acyclovir-resistant HSV infections usually respond to foscarnet (6).

Herpes Varicella-Zoster

Recurrent dermatomal VSV infection (zoster, "shingles") is much more common in HIV-infected patients than in age-matched controls. The typical presentation consists of radicular pain followed by an erythematous rash evolving into fluid-filled vesicles over 1-3 adjacent dermatomes. Widespread cutaneous or visceral dissemination, pneumonia, and hepatitis occasionally occur. Primary infection is rare in adults, but has caused life-threatening illness in immuno-suppressed patients.

Infection of the first branch of cranial nerve V involving the eye (herpes zoster ophthalmicus) usually requires hospitalization. VZV encephalitis is rare, but should be considered in the patient presenting with headache and altered mental status, and possibly cerebellar findings, within 1-12 weeks after onset of localized zoster (1).

Treatment (3,4) of recurrent zoster in HIV-infected patients:
> Acyclovir (Zovirax), 800 mg po 5 times per day for 7-10 days. GI side effects may be more prominent at these doses than when treating for HSV. Primary or disseminated VZV should be treated with acyclovir, 10-12 mg/kg IV, infused over 1 hr, q 8 hrs for 7-14 days (see above for side effects). **Foscarnet appears to be effective in treating acyclovir-resistant VZV (5).**

<u>Suggested Reading</u>
1) Levy RM and DE Bredesen. Central nervous system dysfunction in AIDS. In Rosenblum ML, et al., eds. AIDS and the Nervous System. New York. Raven. 1988.
2) Drew WL, et al. Herpesvirus infections (cytomegalovirus, herpes simplex virus. varicella-zoster virus). How to use ganciclovir (DHPG) and acyclovir. Infectious Disease Clinics of North America 1988; 2:495-509.
3) The Medical Letter on Drugs and Therapeutics. Drugs for AIDS and associated infections. 1991; 33:95-102.
4) The Medical Letter on Drugs and Therapeutics. Drugs for treatment of viral infections. 1992; 34:31-36.
5) Safrin S, et al. Foscarnet therapy in five patients with acyclovir-resistant varicella-zoster infection. Annals of Internal Medicine 1991; 115:19-21.
6) Safrin S, et al. A controlled trial comparing foscarnet with vidarabine for acyclovir-resistant mucocutaneous herpes simplex in the acquired immune deficiency syndrome. NEJM 1991; 325:551-555.

SUMMARY OF AIDS THERAPEUTICS

HIV INFECTION (Antiretroviral therapy)

Zidovudine (AZT, Retrovir)
HIV infected patients with CD4 count <500, or rapidly falling (by >100-150 cells/microliter/year) CD4 count:
200 mg po tid, or 500 mg po per day divided tid (200-100-200).
Post-exposure prophylaxis:
200 mg q 4 hr for 1st 72 hrs, then 100-200 mg 5 times/day for 25 days.

Didanosine (ddl, Videx)
HIV infected patients intolerant to, or deteriorating despite, treatment with AZT; also useful in combination or alternation with AZT:

Weight (kg)	Dose (po)
>75	300 mg bid
50-74	200 mg bid
35-49	125 mg bid

Use at least 2 tablets per dose to provide adequate buffer. Tablets must be crushed or chewed before swallowing.

Zalcitibine (ddC, Hivid)
HIV infected patients deteriorating despite AZT:
0.375 or 0.75 mg po tid, in combination with AZT, 500-600 mg/d.

Combination Therapy: Progression of disease despite AZT. Also, patients presenting initially with opportunistic infection or CD4 count <200 should be begun on combination therapy.

Investigational Drug: Stavudine (d4T)
Available through the manufacturer (Bristol-Meyers-Squib, 1-800-842-8036) for patients failing AZT and DDI.

PNEUMOCYSTIS CARINII PNEUMONIA

SEVERE DISEASE
TMP/SMX, 15 mg TMP/kg/d IV, divided into 3-4 doses per day.

OR

Primaquine, 30 mg base form po qd (each 26 mg primaquine tablet contains 15 mg of base form; dose is therefore 2 tablets),
+ Clindamycin, 450-600 mg IV or po tid.

OR

Pentamidine isethionate, 3-4 mg/kg/d IV as single daily dose.

Some patients (see text) will benefit from adjunctive corticosteroid therapy:
Prednisone (po) or **methylprednisolone** (IV):
Day 1-5: 40 mg bid
Day 6-10: 40 mg qd
Day 11-21: Taper from 20 mg qd to zero.

MILD-TO-MODERATE DISEASE (PaO2 > 70 mm Hg on room air)
TMP/SMX, 2 double-strength tablets po tid-qid.
OR
Trimethoprim, 15 mg/kg/d po, divided into four doses per day,
+ **Dapsone**, 100 mg po qd.

SALVAGE THERAPY (failure of established treatments)
566C80 (Atovaquone), 750 mg po tid (experimental). Available from Burroughs Wellcome (1-800-755-2020).

PROPHYLAXIS (HIV infected patients with CD4 counts < 200, or thrush or severe constitutional symptoms, or prior PCP)
Established:
TMP/SMX, 1 double-strength tablet po qd or three times per week -
OR
Aerosolized Pentamidine, 300 mg q month via Respirgard II jet nebulizer, OR 60 mg 5 times in 1st 2 weeks and 60 mg q 2 wks thereafter via Fisoneb ultrasonic nebulizer. Evidence is accumulating that systemic therapies are in general superior to aerosolized pentamidine.
Investigational:
Dapsone, 50-100 mg po qd, with or without pyrimethamine, 50 mg po q week.
Alternatives: Pyrimethamine/sulfadiazine, pyrimethamine sulfadoxine (Fansidar; potentially fatal Stevens-Johnson syndrome), 566C80 (Atovaquone, experimental), parenteral pentamidine (little data).

TOXOPLASMOSIS

Toxoplasma Encephalitis
Pyrimethamine, 200 mg po 1st day, then 50-100 mg po qd,
AND
Sulfadiazine, 4-6 gm po or IV qd divided into 4 doses per day, OR, if sulfadiazine not tolerated, **Clindamycin**, 450-600 mg po qid, or 600-900 mg IV q 6 hr,
AND **Folinic acid** (leucovorin), 10-50 mg po qd.

Alternative: Pyrimethamine + 566C80 (experimental).

Chronic Suppression
Pyrimethamine, 25 mg po qd,
AND
Sulfadiazine, 500 mg - 1 gm po qid, OR, if sulfadiazine not tolerated, **Clindamycin**, 300 mg po qid,
AND **Folinic acid (leucovorin)**, 10 mg po qd.

Prophylaxis (may be useful in patients with CD4 < 200 and positive toxoplasma titers)
TMP/SMX at PCP prophylaxis doses; other possibilities include pyrimethamine/dapsone, pyrimethamine/sulfadiazine/leucovorin at chronic suppressive doses two days per week, azithromycin, 566C80.

CRYPTOCOCCUS

Severe Pulmonary Disease Same therapy as for high-risk patients with cryptococcal meningitis (see below).
Other Extraneural Cryptococcosis (including positive serum CrAg titer)
Fluconazole, 400 mg po qd.

Cryptococcal Meningitis
High-risk patients (CSF CrAg > 1:1024 OR altered mental status)
Amphotericin B, 0.5-0.8 mg/kg IV qd. In patients with adequate WBC, **Flucytosine**, 25 mg/kg po q 6 hr, may be added.
Low-risk patients (CSF CrAg < 1:1024 AND non-altered mental status)
Fluconazole, 400 mg po qd.
Chronic Suppression
Fluconazole, 200 mg po qd (More effective than weekly amphotericin).

COCCIDIOIDES

Coccidioidomycosis
Established: **Amphotericin B**, 0.5-0.8 mg/kg IV qd, to total dose of 2.5 gm.
Investigational:
Itraconazole (Sporanox), 200 mg po bid, or **Fluconazole**, 200 mg po bid.
Chronic Suppression
Fluconazole, 200 mg po bid,
OR **Amphotericin B**, 1 mg/kg IV q week or biweekly.

HISTOPLASMA

Disseminated Histoplasmosis
Established: **Amphotericin B**, 0.5-0.8 mg/kg IV qd, to total dose of 15 mg/kg.
Investigational:
Itraconazole (Sporanox), 300 mg po bid for 3 days, followed by 200 mg po bid for 12 weeks.
OR **Fluconazole**, 400 mg po bid.

Chronic Suppression
Established: **Amphotericin B**, 1.0 mg/kg q week.
Investigational: **Itraconazole (Sporanox)**, 200 mg po bid.
Anecdotal: Fluconazole, 400 mg po qd.

CANDIDIASIS

Oral Candidiasis
Clotrimazole (Mycelex) troches, 10 mg dissolved in mouth over 15-30 minutes, 3-5 times a day for 2 weeks.
OR
Nystatin (Mycostatin), oral pastilles (200,000 units), one to two dissolved slowly in mouth five times a day; or vaginal tablets
(100,000 U), dissolved slowly in mouth three times a day.
OR
Ketoconazole (Nizoral), 200 mg po qd for two weeks.
OR
Fluconazole (Diflucan), 50-100 mg po qd.

Candida Esophagitis
Fluconazole, 100-200 mg po qd, more effective than **Ketoconazole**, 200-400 mg po qd. Maintenance with fluconazole (100 mg po qd) or ketoconazole (200 mg po qd) may be required.

Candida vaginitis may be treated with commercially available creams or tablets (clotrimazole, nystatin, or miconazole). Ketoconazole, 200 mg po qd for 10 days (see above for precautions), may be used for severe disease. Cures reported with **fluconazole**, 400 mg po as a single dose.

CYTOMEGALOVIRUS

(Dosage adjustments must be made based on creatinine clearance; see text.)

Induction

Ganciclovir (DHPG), 5 mg/kg IV bid for 14-21 days (retinitis) or 21-42 days (gastrointestinal disease),

OR **Foscarnet**, 60 mg/kg IV tid (via infusion pump only) for 14-21 days (retinitis) or 21-42 days (gastrointestinal disease).

Chronic Suppression (following induction for CMV retinitis)

Ganciclovir (DHPG), 5 mg/kg IV qd,

OR **Foscarnet**, 90-120 mg/kg IV qd (via infusion pump only).

HERPES SIMPLEX VIRUS

Primary or Recurrent Mucocutaneous HSV

Acyclovir (Zovirax), 200-400 mg po 5 times a day for 10 days, or 5 mg/kg IV q 8 hr;

OR In cases of acyclovir resistance, **Foscarnet**, 40 mg/kg IV, via infusion pump only, q 8 hr for 21 days.

Visceral Involvement

Acyclovir, 10 mg/kg IV q 8 hr, or possibly **Foscarnet**.

Chronic suppression

Acyclovir, 400 mg po bid;

OR In cases of acyclovir resistance, **Foscarnet**, 40 mg/kg IV, via infusion pump, qd.

VARICELLA ZOSTER VIRUS

Primary or Disseminated Infection

Acyclovir, 10-12 mg/kg IV q 8 hours for 7-14 days;

OR In cases of acyclovir resistance, **Foscarnet**, 40 mg/kg IV, via infusion pump, q 8 hr for 2-4 weeks.

Dermatomal Zoster (Shingles)

Acyclovir, 800 mg po 5 times a day for 7-10 days;

OR In cases of acyclovir resistance, **Foscarnet**, 40 mg/kg IV, via infusion pump, q 8 hr.

MYCOBACTERIUM AVIUM COMPLEX
(Optimal treatment unknown)

One Regimen
Rifampin, 10 mg/kg (max 600 mg) po qd
AND **Ethambutol**, 15-25 mg/kg (max 1000 mg) qd
AND **Clofazamine**, 100 mg po qd
AND **Ciprofloxacin**, 500-750 mg po bid.

Another Regimen
Clarithromycin (Biaxin), 1 gm po bid (If poorly tolerated, lower dose of 500 mg bid may be used),
AND **Ethambutol**, 25 mg/kg po qd
AND **Ciprofloxacin**, 500-750 mg/kg po bid.
(Because of expense, **Clofazamine**, 100 mg po qd, is sometimes substituted for ciprofloxacin in this regimen.)

Amikacin, 10 mg/kg IV qd, may be added in patients who do not respond after 4-6 weeks of oral treatment alone.
Prophylaxis (experimental)
Rifabutin, 300 mg po qd.
Azithromycin and Clarithromycin are also possibly effective.

TUBERCULOSIS

Active Disease
Isoniazid (INH), 300 mg po qd,
AND **Rifampin**, 600 mg po qd,
AND **Pyrazinamide (PZA)**, 15-25 mg/kg qd;
Ethambutol, 15-25 mg/kg qd is added in cases of disseminated or meningeal infection, or suspected INH resistance.
Pyridoxine, 25-50 mg qd should be added to any regimen containing INH.
Three (or four) drug therapy is given for 2 months, with INH and Rifampin continued for a total of 9 months, or 6 months following conversion of cultures to negative, whichever is longer.

Post-exposure prophylaxis (PPD reaction >5 mm, or known exposure to active TB, or anergic patients at high risk)
Isoniazid (INH), 300 mg po qd for one year, plus **pyridoxine**, 25-50 mg po qd.
Drug-Resistant Infection: Consult a TB specialist.

SYPHILIS

Early Disease (Primary, secondary, or latent of < 1 year duration)
Benzathine penicillin, 2.4 million units IM, single injection. Some authorities prefer 3 injections at weekly intervals (7.2 million units total).
Late Latent Disease (Latent > 1 year or unknown duration)
Benzathine penicillin, 2.4 million units IM q week for three doses.

Neurosyphilis
Aqueous penicillin G, 12 million units IV q day for 10 days,

OR

Procaine penicillin, 2.4 million units IM qd for 10 days, plus **probenecid**, 500 mg po qd for 10 days.

Either regimen should be followed by **benzathine penicillin**, 2.4 million units IM q week for 3 weeks.

Investigational: Ceftriaxone, 1 gm IM qd for 10 days.

To Order Additional Copies

Current Clinical Strategies, PSYCHIATRY Lisa Burwell-Sipes	#___x $8.75
Handbook of Psychiatric Drug Therapy Lisa Burwell-Sipes	#___x $8.75
Manual of HIV/AIDS Therapy. Laurence Peiperl	#___x $8.75
Current Clinical Strategies, MEDICINE, Paul D. Chan, NEW 1993 edition	#___x $8.75
Current Clinical Strategies, GYNECOLOGY & OBSTETRICS	#___x $8.75
Current Clinical Strategies, PEDIATRICS	#___x $8.75
FAMILY MEDICINE Pediatrics, Medicine, Gynecology, Obstetrics	#___x $26.25
DIAGNOSTIC HISTORY & PHYSICAL EXAMINATION in MEDICINE	#___x $8.75
OUTPATIENT MEDICINE	#___x $8.75
CRITICAL CARE MEDICINE	#___x $8.75
Current Clinical Strategies, SURGERY (available March 1993)	#___x $8.75
	Total ______

Prices are in US dollars & include shipping; Canada, $10.75; UK, £4.00; Australia, $9.75. Other countries, send equivalent check. Prices and availability subject to change without notice.

Order by Phone: 714-965-9400 (COD orders, add $1.50 per order)

Order by Mail. Send order & check payable to:

Current Clinical Strategies Publishing
9550 Warner Ave, Suite 350
Fountain Valley, Ca USA 92708-2822

Return Address: ____

____

____

Check if Resident or Student ______

Is this book sold at your local medical book store? ___ yes ___ no

Name of bookstore: ____